GREEN SMOOTHIE RECIPES

Luscious Fruit Smoothie Recipes for a Pleasurable and Healthy Summer

(Quick and Healthy Smoothie Recipe for Weight Loss)

Ann Bauer

Published by Alex Howard

© Ann Bauer

All Rights Reserved

Green Smoothie Recipes: Luscious Fruit Smoothie Recipes for a Pleasurable and Healthy Summer (Quick and Healthy Smoothie Recipe for Weight Loss)

ISBN 978-1-990169-82-3

All rights reserved. No part of this guide may be reproduced in any form without permission in writing from the publisher except in the case of brief quotations embodied in critical articles or reviews.

Legal & Disclaimer

The information contained in this book is not designed to replace or take the place of any form of medicine or professional medical advice. The information in this book has been provided for educational and entertainment purposes only.

The information contained in this book has been compiled from sources deemed reliable, and it is accurate to the best of the Author's knowledge; however, the Author cannot guarantee its accuracy and validity and cannot be held liable for any errors or omissions. Changes are periodically made to this book. You must consult your doctor or get professional medical advice before using any of the suggested remedies, techniques, or information in this book.

Table of contents

Part 1 1

Our Skin: From The Inside Out 2

How Smoothies Can Transform Skin 4

How To Combat Oily Skin 5

Citrus Fruit 6

Orange And Lemon Smoothie 6

Grapefruit, Pineapple And Mint Smoothie 7

Orange And Pomegranate Smoothie 8

Mandarin Smoothie 9

Kiwi, Grapefruit And Lime Smoothie 10

Banana Chocolate Smoothie 11

Peanut Butter And Banana Smoothie 12

Banana And Chocolate-Mint Smoothie 13

Banana And Strawberry Smoothie 14

Broccoli And Pineapple Smoothie 15

Mango And Broccoli Smoothie 16

Cherry, Chocolate And Broccoli Smoothie 17

Banana, Cinnamon And Broccoli Smoothie 18

Foods For Total Rehydration 19

Aloe Vera 20

Aloe Vera And Lime Smoothie 21

Aloe Vera, Banana And Blueberry Smoothie 22

Aloe Vera And Honeydew Melon Smoothie 23

Aloe Vera And Pineapple Smoothie 24

Papaya, Lime And Ginger Smoothie 25

Papaya And Pear Smoothie 26

Papaya And Passionfruit Smoothie 27

Papaya And Guava Smoothie 28

How To Calm And Soothe Sensitive Skin 29

Bee Pollen 30

Bee Pollen And Mango Smoothie 30

Bee Pollen And Pineapple Smoothie 31

Bee Pollen, Banana And Avocado Smoothie 32

Peach, Passionfruit And Bee Pollen Smoothie 33

Creamy, Nutty Hemp Smoothie 34

Strawberry And Hemp Smoothie 35

Kiwi, Lime And Hemp Smoothie 36

Beetroot And Hemp Smoothie 37

Turmeric And Ginger Smoothie 38

Turmeric And Berry Smoothie 39

Turmeric And Cherry Smoothie 40

Turmeric And Apricot Smoothie 40

Say Goodbye To Acne-Prone And Problem Skin 41

Carrot And Ginger Smoothie 42

Carrot, Apple And Orange Smoothie ... 43

Carrot, Banana And Beetroot Smoothie ... 44

Carrot And Pear Smoothie ... 45

Green, Cucumber Smoothie ... 46

Cucumber And Kiwi Smoothie ... 47

Cucumber And Pineapple Smoothie ... 48

Cucumber And Nut Butter Smoothie ... 49

Maca, Cacao And Banana Smoothie ... 50

Strawberry And Vanilla Maca Smoothie ... 51

Maca And Cherry Smoothie ... 52

Maca And Goji Berry Smoothie ... 53

How To Make Your Skin Radiate ... 54

Mango And Passionfruit Smoothie ... 55

Mango And Guava Smoothie ... 56

Spinach And Kale ... 57

Spinach And Kale Smoothie ... 57

Super Green Smoothie ... 58

Coconut Water ... 59

Coconut Water, Avocado And Strawberry Smoothie ... 59

Coconut Water, Avocado And Strawberry Smoothie ... 60

Coconut And Lime Smoothie ... 61

Smoothies To Turn Back The Clock ... 62

Chia Seed ... 63

Peanut Butter, Banana And Chia Seed Smoothie 63

Chia Seed And Mango Smoothie 64

Chia And Pomegranate Smoothie 65

Watermelon And Strawberry Smoothie 66

Watermelon, Lime And Mint Smoothie 67

Watermelon And Raspberry Smoothie 68

Royal Jelly 69

Royal Jelly, Mango And Berry Smoothie 70

Royal Jelly, Spinach And Cucumber Smoothie 71

Mint, Blueberry And Royal Jelly Smoothie 72

Strawberry Peanut Butter Banana Smoothie 73

Peanut Butter And Banana Smoothie 74

Chocolate Banana Smoothie 75

Chocolate Peanut Butter Smoothie 76

Nutty Buddy Smoothie 77

Creamy Strawberry Smoothie 78

Orange/Mango Creamy Shake 79

Creamy Choco Almond Shake 80

Creamy Banana Strawberry Shake 81

Peanut Protein Shake 82

Pineapple Coconut Banana Shake 83

Banana Chocolate Malt Shake 84

Chikoo (Sapodilla Fruit) Banana Shake 85

Cookies & Crème Protein Shake 86

Coconut Almond Protein Joy Shake 87

Chia Almond Spinach Shake 88

Double Pina Colada Champion Smoothie 89

Coffee Peanut Protein Dream Smoothie 90

Healthy Weight Gain Smoothie 91

Apple Dates Protein Shake 92

Banana Peanut Protein Shake 93

Albana Blueberry Slurpee Smoothie 94

Strawberry Avocado Smoothie 95

Minty Chocolaty Creamy Shake 96

Sweet Cinnamon Smoothie 97

Strawberry, Banana And Blueberry Smoothie 98

Chocolate Coffee Blend 99

Part 2 100

Banana Smoothie 101

Banana And Strawberry Smoothie 102

Strawberry Shortcake Smoothie 103

Triple Blended Berry Smoothie 104

Orange Raspberry Smoothie 105

Mango Peach Banana Smoothie 106

Almond Honeydew Smoothie 107

Cantaloupe Smoothie 108

- Apple And Carrots Smoothie 109
- Spa Cucumber Smoothie 110
- Cherry Vanilla Smoothie 111
- Grapefruit Smoothie 112
- Ginger Banana Smoothie 113
- Mango Shake 114
- Blue Raspberry Shake 115
- Mixed Berry Shake 116
- Buttermilk Strawberry Shake 117
- Mixed Berry Shake 118
- Cranberry Green Tea Shake 119
- The Energy Shake 120
- Yogurt And Fruit Shake 121
- Mango Blackberry Shake 122
- Strawberry Milk Shake 123
- Fruit Yogurt Shake 124
- Choco Cherry Smoothie 125
- Melon Mint Smoothie 126
- Zinger Ginger Honeydew Smoothie 127
- Guava Smoothie 128
- Cranberry Banana Smoothie 130
- Apricot Berries Smoothie 131
- Pear Blueberry Smoothie 132

Celery Cucumber Smoothie	133
Carrot Celery Ginger Smoothie	134
Turmeric Pineapple Smoothie	136
Cucumber Pineapple Grapefruit Smoothie	138
Turmeric Pumpkin Smoothie	139
Sweet Potato Ginger Smoothie	140
Cucumber Ginger Smoothie	141
Apple Peanut Butter Smoothie	142
Chocolate Avocado Smoothie	143
Hearty Spinach Lentil Soup	144
Yummy Mac And Cheese	146
Creamy And Delicious Potato Mash	147
Kale Lentil Soup	148
Quick And Cheesy Pasta	149
Roasted Potatoes	150
Creamy Mushroom Risotto	151
Quick And Easy Green Beans	153
Delicious Applesauce	153
Easy Steamed Brussels Sprouts	155
Garlic Chickpeas	156
Spinach Squash Risotto	158
Gluten Free Porridge	160
Apple Squash Soup	161

Cilantro Lime Cauliflower Rice 162

Refried Beans 163

Creamy Potato Leek Soup 164

Plain Garlic Rice 165

Red Beans With Rice 166

Quick Sweet Potato Gratin 167

Hot Ginger Carrot Soup 168

Sweet Brown Rice 169

Cilantro Avocado Rice 170

Mushroom Barley Risotto 171

Delicious Sweet Potato Casserole 173

Millet Breakfast Porridge 175

Potato Carrot Corn Chowder 175

Sweet And Spicy Spaghetti 177

Pea Corn Herbed Risotto 178

Healthy Breakfast Quinoa 179

Quick Apple Crisp 180

Garlic Tomato Beans 181

Creamy Squash And Apple Mash 183

Split Pea Curry 184

Part 1

Our Skin: From The Inside Out

As well as being our biggest organ, our skin is our first line of defense. In today's world, skin can define much of our standard for beauty. Youthful, bright skin is associated with health and vitality. It plays an important psychological role as it is our aesthetic. It is what we present to the world; shaping how others see us and how we see ourselves. What we put in our bodies is just as important as our skincare routine.

The skin has three main layers:

Epidermis: The epidermis is our skin's external layer which is visible. This is the part we see, feel and touch. It consists of several layers, and is mostly made up of our dead skin cells.

Dermis: This is the layer that lies underneath the epidermis. The dermis has small blood vessels, nerve endings, oil glands, sweat glands, and hair follicles. It also contains collagen and elastic tissue, which help to keep the skin youthful, firm and strong.

Subcutaneous Layer: Comprised of fat and connective tissue, this layer contains larger blood vessels and nerves. It helps to regulate body and skin temperature.

The skin has its own life cycle. New cells are born at the bottom of the epidermis, and live for 28 days, slowly making their way up until they reach the top layer. They stay on the surface, absorbing moisture and forming the hydro-lipid barrier. Our skin acts as the first physical barrier to protects against wind, cold, pressure, stress or trauma. Our cells are tightly packed against one another and this creates a barricade which prevents the absorption of any external fluid. This allows us to swim, stand in the rain or have a shower without absorbing any water.

We can also block ultraviolet light, which radiates from the sun and would otherwise damage our skin. The melanin in our epidermis is responsible for this. Melanin doesn't offer complete protection, so we should avoid excessive exposure to the sun's rays. The very top layer of our skin is covered with a coat of moisture which prevents us from getting infections. Thermal regulation is yet another thing that our skin does for us. Last but not least, our skin is the main source through which we can absorb vitamin D. When skin is exposed to sunlight, it makes vitamin D from cholesterol.

How Smoothies Can Transform Skin

Beautiful-looking skin starts with the food that we put into our bodies. Fruits and vegetables contain powerful antioxidants which protect our skin from cellular damage. Sun, smoking, pollution and too much sunlight can have negative effects on our skin. By including a rainbow of colorful and fresh food, you can counteract any damage caused.

A smoothie is a mixture of fruits or vegetables pureed in a blender with water, milk or ice. Non-dairy milk is preferable, as dairy can be the cause of many skin problems. Dairy contains natural hormones that can lead to inflammation in the skin. Different to juices, smoothies use the whole ingredient which gives you the added benefit of fiber. Sometimes it can be difficult to include the required daily intake of fruits and vegetables. But by blending everything you need in a cup, you can easily achieve this. As a result, you can increase your vitamin, mineral, and antioxidant intake, and strengthen your immune system.

A vitamin-packed smoothie is a great way to drink your way to better skin. These blends are easy to digest, keep you hydrated, increase your energy levels and can help your skin glow. Your body doesn't need to work hard in order to break down the foods and extract all the goodness. In this e-book we look at the most beneficial smoothies for every type of skin. Keep reading to discover which ones are best for you.

How To Combat Oily Skin

Oily skin occurs when our sebaceous glands produce too much oil. When combined with dead skin, it can clog your pores up and leads to blackheads, whiteheads and breakouts. Other symptoms of oily skin are shiny or greasy appearance, large pores and skin which looks thick or rough.

Citrus Fruit

As well as being very refreshing, citrus fruits are super rich in vitamin C and have detoxifying effects, which will help to flush out any extra oil within the skin.

Orange And Lemon Smoothie

Ingredients:
1 large orange, chopped
¼ lemon
½ cup pineapple, chopped
¼ cup frozen mango, chopped
¼ teaspoon fresh ginger
1 cup unsweetened oat, coconut or nut milk

Directions:
Add all ingredients into a blender, and blend for approximately 1-2 minutes or until smooth. Then pour into a glass and enjoy.

Grapefruit, Pineapple And Mint Smoothie

1 grapefruit
2 cups frozen pineapple, chopped
4 cups spinach leaves
¼ cup chia seeds
½ cup unsweetened oat, coconut or nut milk
¼ teaspoon fresh ginger
2 mint leaves

Directions:

Add all ingredients into a blender, and blend for approximately 1-2 minutes or until smooth. Then pour into a glass and enjoy.

Orange And Pomegranate Smoothie

Ingredients:
1 cup frozen mango, chopped
¼ lemon juice
¼ teaspoon ground cayenne pepper
½ cup freshly squeezed orange juice
2 teaspoons freshly grated ginger
1 small raw, red beet
1 cup frozen raspberries
1 grapefruit, chopped
honey to taste

Directions:
Add all ingredients into a blender, and blend for approximately 1-2 minutes or until smooth. Then pour into a glass and enjoy.

Mandarin Smoothie

4 mandarins
½ cup ice cubes
¼ cup unsweetened oat or nut milk
a pinch of sea salt
1 frozen banana
1 teaspoon freshly grated turmeric or ½ teaspoon ground turmeric
2 drops of vanilla extract

Directions:

Add all ingredients into a blender, and blend for approximately 1-2 minutes or until smooth. Then pour into a glass and enjoy.

Kiwi, Grapefruit And Lime Smoothie

Ingredients:
1 grapefruit, chopped
1 kiwi fruit
2 mandarins
1 pear, chopped
1 ½ tablespoons honey
2 cups ice cubes

Directions:

Add all ingredients into a blender, and blend for approximately 1-2 minutes or until smooth. Then pour into a glass and enjoy.

Banana

Banana is a superior source of phosphates, vitamin D, and potassium. It acts as an excellent skin detoxifier. Banana also help to shrink skin pore size. This is essential in preventing excessive oil secretion and clogging of pores.

Banana Chocolate Smoothie

Ingredients:
1 cup of unsweetened oat, coconut or nut milk
1 frozen banana
2 tablespoons oats
1 teaspoon raw cacao
½ teaspoon cinnamon
½ cup ice cubes
Directions:
Add all ingredients into a blender, and blend for approximately 1-2 minutes or until smooth. Then pour into a glass and enjoy.

Peanut Butter And Banana Smoothie

Ingredients:
½ cup water (or dairy-free milk of choice)
1 frozen banana, cut into pieces
2 tablespoons all-natural peanut butter
1 tablespoon ground flax seeds
½ teaspoon vanilla extract
½ cup ice cubes
Directions:
Add all ingredients into a blender, and blend for approximately 1-2 minutes or until smooth. Then pour into a glass and enjoy.

Banana And Chocolate-Mint Smoothie

Ingredients:
1 cup unsweetened oat, coconut or nut milk
3 cups baby spinach leaves
1 frozen banana
3 tablespoons mint leaves
2 tablespoons flaxseeds
1 cup ice cubes

Directions:
Add all ingredients into a blender, and blend for approximately 1-2 minutes or until smooth. Then pour into a glass and enjoy.

Banana And Strawberry Smoothie

Ingredients:
½ cup frozen blueberries
½ cup frozen raspberries
1 frozen banana
1 cup unsweetened oat, coconut or nut milk
Directions:
Add all ingredients into a blender, and blend for approximately 1-2 minutes or until smooth. Then pour into a glass and enjoy.
Broccoli
As well as being a rich source of Vitamin A and C, broccoli contains properties which are known to reduce the oil production on the skin. This makes it the ideal ingredient for your smoothie. It's most likely not the first choice of ingredient when you think about making a smoothie. The smoothies below take away any bitterness from the broccoli and are absolutely delicious.

Broccoli And Pineapple Smoothie

Ingredients:
1 cup broccoli florets
1 ½ cups pineapple, chopped
1 frozen banana
1-2 cups fresh baby spinach leaves
1 cup unsweetened oat, coconut or nut milk
Directions:
Add all ingredients into a blender, and blend for approximately 1-2 minutes or until smooth. Then pour into a glass and enjoy.

Mango And Broccoli Smoothie

Ingredients:
½ cup raw broccoli florets
1 frozen banana
1 cup frozen mango
½ cup strawberries, fresh or frozen
½ cup spinach leaves
1 cup water
Directions:
Add all ingredients into a blender, and blend for approximately 1-2 minutes or until smooth. Then pour into a glass and enjoy.

Cherry, Chocolate And Broccoli Smoothie

Ingredients:

2 cups water

¼ cup walnuts (you can soak these overnight if you find nuts hard on the stomach)

1 cup frozen cherries

2 cups frozen broccoli florets

1 frozen banana

1 tablespoon raw cacao powder

2 large dates, pitted

1 drop of vanilla extract

Directions:

Add all ingredients into a blender, and blend for approximately 1-2 minutes or until smooth. Then pour into a glass and enjoy.

Banana, Cinnamon And Broccoli Smoothie

Ingredients:
1 ½ cups unsweetened oat, coconut or nut milk
1 frozen banana
2 cups frozen broccoli florets
1 teaspoon ground cinnamon
1 tablespoon honey or maple syrup
Directions:
Add all ingredients into a blender, and blend for approximately 1-2 minutes or until smooth. Then pour into a glass and enjoy.

Foods For Total Rehydration

Healthy skin is smooth, soft and has a strong moisture barrier. This barrier serves as a protective layer and keeps skin hydrated. When this barrier is damaged, it leads to dry skin. Dry skin lacks sebum. the lack of oil leaves it looking flakey and bumpy, sometimes leading to red patches. It can feel itchy, rough, tight and scaly. Transform your dry and irritated skin, and replace it with skin that feels soft and supple. Try out the moisture-boosting smoothies below, and you'll begin to notice the changes.

Aloe Vera

The aloe plant is water-dense, so it's a fantastic way to treat dehydrated skin. This hydrating plant is a rich source of antioxidants and vitamins which protect the skin. Containing vitamins A, C, E, B1, B2, B3 and B6, you can see why it is a superfood! It may also help reduce skin conditions like psoriasis and dermatitis.

When using fresh aloe vera from a plant, trim the ends and remove all of the prickly bits from the plant. Filet each piece of aloe vera by cutting it vertically down the middle. Scoop the fleshy gel with a spoon, being careful not to include any of the green or yellow parts from the leaf. Transfer the gel to your blender. If you don't have an aloe vera plant, you can substitute this for aloe vera juice which is sold in any good health food store.

Aloe Vera And Lime Smoothie

Ingredients:
¼ cup fresh aloe gel
1 cup filtered water
1 cups frozen strawberries
1 ½ tablespoon maple syrup
1 tablespoon lime juice
Directions:
Add all ingredients into a blender, and blend for approximately 1-2 minutes or until smooth. Then pour into a glass and enjoy.

Aloe Vera, Banana And Blueberry Smoothie

Ingredients:
¼ cup fresh aloe gel
½ cup unsweetened oat, coconut or nut milk
1 banana
2 cups frozen blueberries
1 tablespoon ground flaxseed meal
1 tablespoon almond butter
¼ teaspoon cinnamon

Directions:
Add all ingredients into a blender, and blend for approximately 1-2 minutes or until smooth. Then pour into a glass and enjoy.

Aloe Vera And Honeydew Melon Smoothie

Ingredients:
2 cups honeydew melon
4 tablespoons fresh aloe vera
1 apple
¼ teaspoon lime zest
1 ½ cups ice cubes
¼ teaspoon salt

Directions:
Add all ingredients into a blender, and blend for approximately 1-2 minutes or until smooth. Then pour into a glass and enjoy.

Aloe Vera And Pineapple Smoothie

Ingredients:
½ cup frozen pineapple, chopped
1 tablespoon ground flaxseed
2 tablespoons freshly grated ginger
1 cup frozen or fresh spinach
4 tablespoons fresh aloe vera
4-5 ice cubes
4-5 blackberries
Directions:
Add all ingredients into a blender, and blend for approximately 1-2 minutes or until smooth. Then pour into a glass and enjoy.

Papaya

The papaya is a tropical fruit and is grown in hot climates. It can have natural painkiller properties because of the enzyme papain. This enzyme increases the body's production of cytokines, which are a group of proteins that help regulate inflammation. It is very rich in vitamin A as well as enzymes. The vitamin A exfoliates and gets rid of dead skin cells, reducing dryness and giving you a beautiful, natural glow.

Papaya, Lime And Ginger Smoothie

Ingredients:
1 ½ cups frozen papaya, chopped
1 frozen banana
1-2 teaspoons freshly grated ginger
2 freshly squeezed limes
1 cup of unsweetened oat, coconut or nut milk
Directions:
Add all ingredients into a blender, and blend for approximately 1-2 minutes or until smooth. Then pour into a glass and enjoy.

Papaya And Pear Smoothie

Ingredients:
1 frozen papaya, chopped
1 pear, chopped
½ freshly squeezed lime
3 dates, pitted
3 tablespoons coconut milk
pinch of sea salt
1 teaspoon honey
1 cup water
4 ice cubes
Directions:
Add all ingredients into a blender, and blend for approximately 1-2 minutes or until smooth. Then pour into a glass and enjoy.

Papaya And Passionfruit Smoothie

Ingredients:
½ medium papaya
1 banana
4 ripe passion fruits
1 ½ cups unsweetened oat, coconut or nut milk
½ teaspoon ground turmeric
1 tablespoon lime juice
2 tablespoons honey
1 cup ice cubes

Directions:
Add all ingredients into a blender, and blend for approximately 1-2 minutes or until smooth. Then pour into a glass and enjoy.

Papaya And Guava Smoothie

Ingredients:
1 cup papaya, chopped
2-3 small guavas
1 sprig parsley
1 tablespoon lemon juice
½ teaspoon freshly grated ginger
1 teaspoon honey or maple syrup
3-4 ice cubes

Directions:

Add all ingredients into a blender, and blend for approximately 1-2 minutes or until smooth. Then pour into a glass and enjoy.

How To Calm And Soothe Sensitive Skin

Sensitive skin is the result of the nerve endings in the upper layer of the skin becoming irritated. The extremeness of skin sensitivity can vary from an occasional reaction, to full on flare-ups with severe sensitivity every single day. This can result in blemishes, redness, and dry, flakey patches.. In order to prevent this, it is important to focus on soothing, calming fruits and supplements. These create strong barriers so the defenses are not compromised.

Bee Pollen

Bee pollen granules are packed with nutrients and are one of the best foods for your skin. Bee pollen is a complete protein source and contains twenty-two amino acids which are vital for the production of new skin cells. Bee pollen is also an excellent source of energy-boosting B complex vitamins. It is often used as a remedy for allergies, since it contains the anti-histaminic phytochemical quercetin.

Bee Pollen And Mango Smoothie

Ingredients:
½ cup of frozen mango
1-2 tablespoons bee pollen
1 tablespoon honey
1 banana
¼ teaspoon cardamom
¼ teaspoon cinnamon
½ teaspoon turmeric
1 pinch of pepper
Directions:
Add all ingredients into a blender, and blend for approximately 1-2 minutes or until smooth. Then pour into a glass and enjoy.

Bee Pollen And Pineapple Smoothie

Ingredients:
1 banana
½ peach, chopped
½ cup pineapple, chopped
½ cup unsweetened oat, coconut or nut milk
2 ice cubes
1 teaspoon bee pollen
optional: juice of ½ grapefruit, if you like sour citrus
Directions:
Add all ingredients into a blender, and blend for approximately 1-2 minutes or until smooth. Then pour into a glass and enjoy.

Bee Pollen, Banana And Avocado Smoothie

Ingredients:
2 cups spinach leaves
½ avocado, chopped
1 frozen banana
½ freshly squeezed lemon
1 teaspoon bee pollen
1 cup water
2-3 pitted dates or a teaspoon of honey (optional)
4 ice cubes

Directions:

Add all ingredients into a blender, and blend for approximately 1-2 minutes or until smooth. Then pour into a glass and enjoy.

Peach, Passionfruit And Bee Pollen Smoothie

Ingredients:
2 bananas
1 teaspoon freshly grated ginger
3 kiwi fruits, chopped
1 cup of unsweetened oat, coconut or nut milk
1 teaspoon honey (optional)
4 ice cubes

Directions:

Add all ingredients into a blender, and blend for approximately 1-2 minutes or until smooth. Then pour into a glass and enjoy.

Hemp

Hemp provides a complete source of protein which support cell building and repair, for healthier skin, hair, and nails. Hemp contains all 21 known amino acids, including the nine essential amino acids that the body can't produce on its own, all of which your body needs to heal and produce new skin cells. It's also a great source of omega fatty acids, which are anti-inflammatory and anti-aging. The gamma-linolenic acid within hemp is an important fat for good, healthy skin and can even help the healing of eczema. With the added bonus of fiber, iron and zinc, it's the perfect remedy for boosting a healthy complexion.

Creamy, Nutty Hemp Smoothie

Ingredients:
¼ cup hemp seeds
1 cup unsweetened oat, coconut or nut milk
1 frozen banana
1 cup frozen strawberries
1 teaspoon vanilla extract
1 teaspoon cinnamon
2-3 pitted dates for added sweetness (optional)
Directions:
Add all ingredients into a blender, and blend for approximately 1-2 minutes or until smooth. Then pour into a glass and enjoy.

Strawberry And Hemp Smoothie

Ingredients
10 frozen strawberries
1 frozen banana
1 cup unsweetened oat, coconut or nut milk
¼ cup hemp seeds
½ teaspoon vanilla extract
Directions:
Add all ingredients into a blender, and blend for approximately 1-2 minutes or until smooth. Then pour into a glass and enjoy.

Kiwi, Lime And Hemp Smoothie

Ingredients:
2 ice cubes
1 ½ cup unsweetened oat, coconut or nut milk
2 kiwi fruits
2 tablespoons lime juice
1 cup kale
2 tablespoons chia seeds
1 tablespoon hemp seeds
Directions:
Add all ingredients into a blender, and blend for approximately 1-2 minutes or until smooth. Then pour into a glass and enjoy.

Beetroot And Hemp Smoothie

Ingredients:
1 tablespoon hemp seeds
1 small raw, peeled beetroot
1 large apple, chopped
1 stalk of celery, chopped
1 cup unsweetened oat, coconut or nut milk
½ cup frozen peaches
1 teaspoon freshly grated ginger
Directions:
Add all ingredients into a blender, and blend for approximately 1-2 minutes or until smooth. Then pour into a glass and enjoy.

Turmeric

Turmeric is beneficial for all skin types, but it's especially helpful for anyone suffering from psoriasis, irritated or sensitive skin. Turmeric combats redness, puffiness, or scarring by soothing the inflammation. Turmeric contains the chemical curcumin. Curcumin and other chemicals in turmeric have anti-inflammatory properties and can decrease swelling and inflammation.

Turmeric And Ginger Smoothie

Ingredients:
1 cup unsweetened oat, coconut or nut milk
1 mango, chopped
1 cup pineapple, chopped
1 frozen banana
1 teaspoon freshly grated ginger
1 teaspoon freshly grated turmeric or ½ teaspoon ground turmeric
Directions:
Add all ingredients into a blender, and blend for approximately 1-2 minutes or until smooth. Then pour into a glass and enjoy.

Turmeric And Berry Smoothie

Ingredients:
1 cup of unsweetened oat, coconut or nut milk
2 cups baby spinach leaves
3 tablespoons oats
1 cup frozen mixed berries
1½ teaspoons freshly grated turmeric
2 tablespoons honey
1½ teaspoons freshly grated ginger
Directions:
Add all ingredients into a blender, and blend for approximately 1-2 minutes or until smooth. Then pour into a glass and enjoy.

Turmeric And Cherry Smoothie

2 cups frozen cherries
1 cup frozen blueberries
1 frozen banana, chopped
1 teaspoon freshly grated turmeric or ½ teaspoon ground turmeric
2 cups dark leafy greens (spinach or kale)
1 cup unsweetened oat, coconut or nut milk
4 tablespoons hemp seeds
Directions:
Add all ingredients into a blender, and blend for approximately 1-2 minutes or until smooth. Then pour into a glass and enjoy.

Turmeric And Apricot Smoothie

Ingredients:
1 teaspoon freshly grated turmeric
1 cup apricots
1 cup unsweetened oat, coconut or nut milk
2 teaspoons honey
1 cup frozen strawberries
Directions:
Add all ingredients into a blender, and blend for approximately 1-2 minutes or until smooth. Then pour into a glass and enjoy.

Say Goodbye To Acne-Prone And Problem Skin

Blemish-prone skin produces comedones and pimples, is often oily, and appears shiny. This is because more sebum is produced than in other skin types. Painful acne lesions can form, leading to conditions such as cystic acne. These large, red breakouts are deep in your skin and can result in scarring.

Interestingly, those with acne problems have been shown to have vitamin E, A, and zinc deficiencies. Below are some vitamin-packed smoothies to help you combat breakouts and clear your complexion.

Carrots

Carrots are best known for their ability to improve and protect eyesight. The health benefits of eating carrots extend to the skin. If your skin is suffering from dullness or is showing signs of ageing, you can use carrots to coax out your skin's natural glow. Carrots also have an exceptional amount of vitamin A, which helps to slough away old skin cells and regenerate the skin. They can also help with external signs of aging caused by harmful free radicals, as they contain a substance called retinoic acid, which appears to aid the body in maintaining healthy skin.

Carrot And Ginger Smoothie

Ingredients:
1 cup ice cubes
½ cup freshly squeezed orange juice
½ cup sliced carrots
1 teaspoon freshly grated ginger
1 tablespoon lemon juice
1 teaspoon honey (optional)

Directions:

Add all ingredients into a blender, and blend for approximately 1-2 minutes or until smooth. Then pour into a glass and enjoy.

Carrot, Apple And Orange Smoothie

Ingredients:
2 apples, chopped
3 frozen oranges, chopped
1 cup water
½ teaspoon freshly grated ginger
1 teaspoon freshly grated turmeric or ½ teaspoon ground turmeric
a pinch of cayenne pepper
Directions:
Add all ingredients into a blender, and blend for approximately 1-2 minutes or until smooth. Then pour into a glass and enjoy.

Carrot, Banana And Beetroot Smoothie

Ingredients:
2 raw beets, peeled and chopped
2 frozen oranges
3 medium carrots, chopped
1 teaspoon freshly grated ginger
1 cup water
1 frozen banana, chopped

Directions:
Add all ingredients into a blender, and blend for approximately 1-2 minutes or until smooth. Then pour into a glass and enjoy.

Carrot And Pear Smoothie

Ingredients:
1 raw beet, peeled and chopped
1 apple
1 tablespoon of freshly grated ginger
3 carrots, chopped
1 apple, chopped
4 ice cubes

Directions:
Add all ingredients into a blender, and blend for approximately 1-2 minutes or until smooth. Then pour into a glass and enjoy.

Cucumber

With their high water content, cucumbers are excellent for hydration. Not only that; but they are also incredibly anti-inflammatory. They reduce redness, skin irritation and flakiness. High in silica; they have very positive effects on the skin's appearance. Not only that, but thanks to the anti-inflammatory phytonutrients they contain, cucumbers are also great for reducing redness and other skin irritations.

Green, Cucumber Smoothie

Ingredients:
1 cucumber, chopped
¼ cup mint leaves
1 green apple, chopped
1 tablespoon honey
½ avocado, chopped
1 cup ice cubes

Directions:

Add all ingredients into a blender, and blend for approximately 1-2 minutes or until smooth. Then pour into a glass and enjoy.

Cucumber And Kiwi Smoothie

Ingredients:
1 cucumber, chopped
1 kiwi fruit, chopped
1 green apple, chopped
1 cup coconut water
½ teaspoon lemon juice
4 mint leaves
1 teaspoon chia seeds
1 cup ice cubes

Directions:
Add all ingredients into a blender, and blend for approximately 1-2 minutes or until smooth. Then pour into a glass and enjoy.

Cucumber And Pineapple Smoothie

Ingredients:

½ cup cucumber, chopped

1 cup frozen pineapple, chopped

½ frozen banana, chopped

½ cup coconut milk

½ cup water

1 lime, juiced

1 cup of leafy greens (spinach or kale)

2-4 ice cubes

Directions:

Add all ingredients into a blender, and blend for approximately 1-2 minutes or until smooth. Then pour into a glass and enjoy.

Cucumber And Nut Butter Smoothie

Ingredients:

½ cucumber, chopped

1 medium pear, chopped

1 tablespoon almond butter or other nut butter of your choice

1 tablespoon chia seeds

1 teaspoon cinnamon

1 cup unsweetened oat, coconut or nut milk

6 ice cubes

Directions:

Add all ingredients into a blender, and blend for approximately 1-2 minutes or until smooth. Then pour into a glass and enjoy.

Maca

Maca is a superfood and is believed to improve fertility, boost libido, sharpen mental focus, help memory, enhance endurance, reduce the symptoms of menopause, and more. Known for assisting with hormonal problems, it aids in bringing the system back into balance. It helps to clear blemishes and acne, and fast-tracks collagen production. Maca is full of vitamins, including B1, B2, C, and E. It also contains calcium, zinc, iron, and essential amino acids. It adds a caramel or malt-like taste to your smoothies.

Maca, Cacao And Banana Smoothie

Ingredients:

1 cup unsweetened oat, coconut or nut milk

1 frozen banana, chopped

1 tablespoon maca powder

½ tablespoon cacao powder

5 ice cubes

Directions:

Add all ingredients into a blender, and blend for approximately 1-2 minutes or until smooth. Then pour into a glass and enjoy.

Strawberry And Vanilla Maca Smoothie

Ingredients:
1 frozen banana, chopped
1 cup strawberries
1 cup unsweetened oat, coconut or nut milk
1 tablespoon maca powder
4 to 6 ice cubes

Directions:
Add all ingredients into a blender, and blend for approximately 1-2 minutes or until smooth. Then pour into a glass and enjoy.

Maca And Cherry Smoothie

Ingredients:

3 cups unsweetened oat, coconut or nut milk

3 cups frozen cherries

2 bananas, chopped

1 teaspoon maca powder

2 teaspoon raw cacao powder

4 to 6 ice cubes

Directions:

Add all ingredients into a blender, and blend for approximately 1-2 minutes or until smooth. Then pour into a glass and enjoy.

Maca And Goji Berry Smoothie

Ingredients:
3 cups unsweetened oat, coconut or nut milk
½ cup goji berries
1 tablespoon raw cacao powder
1 tablespoon maca powder
½ cup frozen blueberries
1 fresh or frozen banana, chopped
a pinch of salt

Directions:
Add all ingredients into a blender, and blend for approximately 1-2 minutes or until smooth. Then pour into a glass and enjoy.

How To Make Your Skin Radiate

We all crave luminous and dewy skin. Our skin is constantly shedding dead skin cells, and if it isn't working efficiently, your complexion can take on a dull, unhealthy, lifeless appearance which can emphasize wrinkles.

Everyday living can cause our skin to become lackluster as it breathes in the everyday pollution we are exposed to. But you can turn this around by adding some key ingredients to your smoothies. Achieve a luminous glow by ensuring you are getting the nutrients you need to let your skin shine.

Mango

Mangoes are not only delicious, but they contain carotenoids, which help our skin glow. Rich in beta-carotene and vitamin A, these carotenoids enrich skin health. Beta-carotene is also a photo-protective agent, protecting the skin from harmful ultraviolet rays.

Mango And Passionfruit Smoothie

Ingredients:

1 frozen mango, chopped

2 passion fruits

1 frozen banana, chopped

1 peach, chopped

1 cup unsweetened oat, coconut or nut milk

Directions:

Add all ingredients into a blender, and blend for approximately 1-2 minutes or until smooth. Then pour into a glass and enjoy.

Mango And Guava Smoothie

Ingredients:
1 cup strawberries
¾ cup mango frozen, chopped
1 banana
¾ cup guava, chopped
1 cup water
1 tablespoon ground flaxseed

Directions:
Add all ingredients into a blender, and blend for approximately 1-2 minutes or until smooth. Then pour into a glass and enjoy.

Spinach And Kale

Green smoothies are incredibly nutrient-dense and they include vegetables that most of us just don't eat enough of - dark leafy greens! They are antioxidant-rich, high in vitamin C, and extremely potent. Not only do they brighten skin, they also reduce inflammation and help to improve skin texture and skin tone.

Spinach And Kale Smoothie

Ingredients:
1 handful kale leaves
1 handful baby spinach leaves
½ cup frozen blueberries
1 cup unsweetened oat, coconut or nut milk
 8 raw almonds
1 tablespoon of spirulina powder
1 teaspoon cinnamon
Directions:
Add all ingredients into a blender, and blend for approximately 1-2 minutes or until smooth. Then pour into a glass and enjoy.

Super Green Smoothie

Ingredients:

½ ripe avocado

1 frozen banana, chopped

1 cup fresh or frozen mixed berries

2 large handfuls spinach leaves

1 small handful kale leaves

1 cup unsweetened oat, coconut or nut milk

1 tablespoon ground flaxseed

2 tablespoons salted almond or peanut butter

Directions:

Add all ingredients into a blender, and blend for approximately 1-2 minutes or until smooth. Then pour into a glass and enjoy.

Coconut Water

Besides being absolutely delicious, coconut water is very hydrating and remineralizing; making our skin look more youthful and supple. The electrolytes in coconut water are comparable to our own blood plasma. Drinking plenty of coconut water rehydrates the skin, giving it a healthy and plump look. With its sweet taste, it's the perfect addition to a smoothie.

Coconut Water, Avocado And Strawberry Smoothie

Ingredients:
1 ½ cups coconut water
1 avocado, chopped
1 cup carrots, chopped
1 cup frozen strawberries
1 cup frozen mango, chopped
Directions:
Add all ingredients into a blender, and blend for approximately 1-2 minutes or until smooth. Then pour into a glass and enjoy.

Coconut Water, Avocado And Strawberry Smoothie

Ingredients:

1 freshly squeezed lime

1 apple, chopped

1 cucumber, chopped

½ cup kale leaves

½ cup spinach leaves

1 teaspoon freshly grated ginger

2 cups coconut water

Directions:

Add all ingredients into a blender, and blend for approximately 1-2 minutes or until smooth. Then pour into a glass and enjoy.

Coconut And Lime Smoothie

Ingredients:

1 ½ cups spinach leaves

2 cups pineapple, chopped

1 banana, chopped

1 freshly juiced lime

½ cup of coconut milk

1-2 teaspoons honey

½ cup of water

5-6 ice cubes

Directions:

Add all ingredients into a blender, and blend for approximately 1-2 minutes or until smooth. Then pour into a glass and enjoy.

Smoothies To Turn Back The Clock

Skin aging is inevitable, but lifestyle and environmental factors can make us appear older than we are. As we age, we lose elastic tissue, our collagen decreases and our epidermis becomes thinner, with the skin eventually ending up more fragile. But we can slow the acceleration of aging and help our skin appear more youthful by consuming collagen-boosting foods.

Chia Seed

Chia seeds are a top-shelf smoothie ingredient. They provide one of the richest sources of omega-3 fatty acids. Omega-3 fatty acids help provide building blocks for healthy skin, cell function and new collagen production, helping minimize wrinkles and fine lines.

Peanut Butter, Banana And Chia Seed Smoothie

Ingredients:
1 banana, chopped
3 tablespoons peanut butter
2 cups unsweetened oat, coconut or nut milk
2 tablespoons chia seeds
1 teaspoon honey (optional)
Directions:
Add all ingredients into a blender, and blend for approximately 1-2 minutes or until smooth. Then pour into a glass and enjoy.

Chia Seed And Mango Smoothie

Ingredients:
1 frozen mango, chopped
½ cup fresh mango, chopped
1 frozen banana, chopped
½ cup nut milk
1 tablespoon nut butter of your choice
2 teaspoons maca root powder
1 teaspoon freshly grated turmeric, or ½ teaspoon of ground turmeric
1 tablespoon chia seed

Directions:
Add all ingredients into a blender, and blend for approximately 1-2 minutes or until smooth. Then pour into a glass and enjoy.

Chia And Pomegranate Smoothie

Ingredients:

1 cup pomegranate seeds

1 banana, chopped

2 cups unsweetened oat, coconut or nut milk

1 tablespoon chia seeds

1 tablespoon ground flax seeds

4 dates, pitted

dash of cinnamon

Directions:

Add all ingredients into a blender, and blend for approximately 1-2 minutes or until smooth. Then pour into a glass and enjoy.

Watermelon

If your skin is showing signs of sun damage, dark spots or premature aging, then it's time to start adding this vitamin-rich fruit to your smoothies, in order to fast-track healing. The combination of vitamin A and C that watermelon possesses helps to restore skin damage caused by exposure to the elements and stress. The vitamin E that watermelon contains can also actually fill out fine lines and lighten the skin.

Watermelon And Strawberry Smoothie

Ingredients:

1 ½ cups fresh watermelon, chopped

1 cup frozen strawberries

½ frozen banana

½ cup unsweetened oat, coconut or nut milk

1 freshly squeezed lemon

1 tablespoon chia or hemp seeds

Directions:

Add all ingredients into a blender, and blend for approximately 1-2 minutes or until smooth. Then pour into a glass and enjoy.

Watermelon, Lime And Mint Smoothie

Ingredients:

3 cups watermelon, chopped

2 tablespoons freshly squeezed lime juice

5 fresh mint leaves

Directions: Blend all ingredients for approximately 1-2 minutes or until smooth. Then pour into a glass and enjoy.

Watermelon And Raspberry Smoothie

Ingredients:

1 cup unsweetened oat, coconut or nut milk

3 cups watermelon, chopped

2 cups raspberries

6 fresh mint leaves

1 cup ice cubes

Directions:

Add all ingredients into a blender, and blend for approximately 1-2 minutes or until smooth. Then pour into a glass and enjoy.

Royal Jelly

Royal jelly is what worker bees feed the queen bee - and it must be pretty potent stuff, considering that worker bees live for seven weeks, whereas the queen bee lives for seven years! Royal jelly is thought to have anti-aging effects, and is packed with nutrients and proteins which are excellent for skin health and elasticity.

Royal Jelly, Mango And Berry Smoothie

Ingredients:

4 teaspoons ground flax seed

1 teaspoon bee pollen

1 teaspoon royal jelly

2 cups unsweetened oat, coconut or nut milk

1 banana, chopped

1 mango, chopped

½ cup frozen strawberries

8 frozen blackberries

8 frozen raspberries

Directions:

Add all ingredients into a blender, and blend for approximately 1-2 minutes or until smooth. Then pour into a glass and enjoy.

Royal Jelly, Spinach And Cucumber Smoothie

Ingredients:
1 handful spinach leaves
1 handful kale leaves
1 cucumber, chopped
1 cup frozen grapes
½ avocado, chopped
2 tablespoons almond butter
½ cup basil
½ cup fresh mint leaves
1 teaspoon royal jelly
1 cup coconut water
Directions:
Add all ingredients into a blender, and blend for approximately 1-2 minutes or until smooth. Then pour into a glass and enjoy.

Mint, Blueberry And Royal Jelly Smoothie

Ingredients:

1 teaspoon royal jelly

½ cup mint leaves

½ cup frozen blueberries

½ cup frozen strawberries

2 bananas, chopped

1 cup unsweetened oat, coconut or nut milk

1 freshly squeezed lemon

¼ teaspoon vanilla extract

9 ice cubes

Directions:

Add all ingredients into a blender, and blend for approximately 1-2 minutes or until smooth. Then pour into a glass and enjoy.

Strawberry Peanut Butter Banana Smoothie

Ingredients
- 3/4 Cup Plain Yogurt
- 5 large frozen Strawberries
- 1 Banana
- 2 Tbsp Peanut Butter
- 2 Tbsp Milk (a splash)

Directions

1. Add milk, yogurt and banana in a blender followed by peanut butter and frozen strawberries.
2. **Blend until it becomes a thick consistency paste, if you like smoothie thinner, add more milk.**
3. You can replace your smooth peanut butter with a crunchy one if you wish to add some crunch to it.

Peanut Butter And Banana Smoothie

Ingredients
- 3/4 Cup plain or vanilla yogurt
- 2 Tbs Peanut Butter
- 1 Banana
- 1/8 Cup milk
- 3/4 Cup ice

Directions
1. Put milk, yogurt and banana in a blender and make smooth consistency paste.
2. **Add crunchy or smooth peanut butter to it and blend further.**
3. You can add desired amount of ice as per your preference.

Chocolate Banana Smoothie

Ingredients
- ¼ Cup milk
- ¾ Cup plain or vanilla yogurt
- 1 Banana
- 3 Dove Chocolates (dark) or roughly 2-3 Tbsp Chips
- 1 Cup ice

Directions
1. Pour milk in a blender followed by banana, chocolate, and yogurt.
2. **Blend until it becomes smooth in consistency.**
3. Add ice and blend again, if you like to have chunks of chocolate then stop blending when its still coarse.

Chocolate Peanut Butter Smoothie

Ingredients
- ¼ Cup milk
- ¾ Cup plain or vanilla yogurt
- 1 Banana
- 2-3 Tbsp Dark Chocolate Chips
- 1 Cup ice
- 2 Tbsp Peanut Butter

Directions
1. Pour the milk in the blender, add yogurt, banana and chocolate to it.
2. Once its blended in smooth mix, add peanut butter and ice to it and blend it again until there are no ice and chocolate chunks left.

Nutty Buddy Smoothie

Ingredients
- 1 Cup Milk
- 1 Ripe Banana
- 1/4 Cup Mixed Nuts
- 2 Tbsp Peanut butter
- 2 Scoop Whey protein powder
- 2 Tsp Honey
- 1 Tsp Cocoa powder

Directions
1. Put milk and banana in blender to form a smooth paste, add mixed nuts like cashews, almonds, peanuts, pistachios to it and blend again.
2. **Add whey protein and blend again until it blends well with the smoothie.**
3. Now add flavor in the form of honey and cocoa powder and blend again.
4. You can also sprinkle some cinnamon or nutmeg powder for added flavor.

Creamy Strawberry Smoothie

Ingredients
- 1-2 cups fresh strawberry
- 1 cup frozen banana
- ⅓ cup of cashews
- 3 pitted dates
- 2 tbsp. vanilla protein
- Almond milk to fill line

Directions
1. Put all the ingredients in a blender at once and blend them until they turn into a smooth paste. If the consistency is too thick.
2. **Add more of almond milk to it.**
3. Add ice to chill it to beat the summer heat.

Orange/Mango Creamy Shake

Ingredients
- Orange/Mango juice 200 ml
- Full-fat milk 200 ml
- Milk cream 100 ml
- Protein powder 2 full scoops
- Ice cubes, a few
- A small banana
- 1 tablespoon honey

Directions
1. Place all in a blender and give it a whirl till smooth.
2. Adjust ice cubes for thickness of the liquid.

Creamy Choco Almond Shake

Ingredients
- Full-fat milk 400 ml
- Chocolate bar 50 gm
- Milk Cream 50 gms
- Almond powder/butter 50 gms
- Coarsely grated almond 1 tablespoon
- Protein powder 2 full scoops
- Ice cubes
- Honey 1 tablespoon
- 1 small banana

Directions
1. Mash banana, honey, cream, protein powder and chocolate and blend in a mixer for a minute or until smooth.
2. Add milk and ice and blend again till a thick cream textured shake results.
3. Add grated almonds for that crunchy flavor.

Creamy Banana Strawberry Shake

Ingredients
- Strawberries 6-8
- Banana 1 big
- Strawberry ice cream 1 big cup
- Full-fat milk 400 ml
- Protein powder 2 full scoops
- Milk cream 50 ml
- Honey 1 tablespoon
- Coarsely ground chocolate chips 2 tablespoon
- Ice cubes

Directions
1. Blend strawberries and banana first.
2. Add honey, cream, protein powder and some milk and blend again.
3. Add balance milk and ice and blend again till a thick creamy shake is obtained.
   4. Sprinkle chocolate chips.

Peanut Protein Shake

Ingredients

- Roasted peanuts coarsely grated 50 gms
- Banana 1 big
- Milk cream 70 ml
- Full-fat milk 400 ml
- Almond butter 1 tablespoon
- Strawberries 6-8
- Protein powder 2 full scoops
- Honey 1 tablespoon
- Ice cubes

Directions

1. Blend almond butter, cream, strawberries and protein powder.
2. Add banana and honey and blend again.
3. Now add milk, ice cubes and peanuts and give it a whirl.

Pineapple Coconut Banana Shake

Ingredients

- Coconut cream 100 ml
- Coconut water 50 ml
- Pineapple slices 4
- Banana 1 small
- Full-fat milk 400 ml
- Milk cream 50 ml
- Protein scoop 2 full scoops
- Ice cubes

Directions

1. Blend all creams, coconut water and pineapple in a smooth paste.
2. Add banana, protein scoop and milk and again blend.
3. Now add ice and give it a whirl.

Banana Chocolate Malt Shake

Ingredients
- Curd (dahi) 100 gms
- Banana 1 large
- Chocolate powder 1 tablespoon
- Any malt based energy drink powder 2 tablespoons
- Full-fat milk 400 ml
- Cream 100 ml
- Honey 2 tablespoons
- Whey protein powder 2 scoops
- Ice cubes

Directions
1. Blend banana, cream, honey and protein powder first.
2. Add the rest and blend.
3. Add ice and give it a whirl.

Chikoo (Sapodilla Fruit) Banana Shake

Ingredients
- Chikoo 2 big
- Banana 1 small
- Milk 400 ml
- Vanilla ice cream 1 cup big
- Honey 1 tablespoon
- Whey protein 2 scoops
- Peanut roasted and grated coarsely 1 tablespoon
- **Ice**

Directions
1. Blend Chikoo and Banana and ice cream together.
2. Add protein powder, milk and honey and blend till smooth.
3. Now add ice and give it a final whirl.

Cookies & Crème Protein Shake

Ingredients
- 1 scoop cookies and crème protein powder
- 2 cups almond milk
- 4 tablespoons drinking chocolate
- 50 ml whipped cream
- 1 cup broken ice
- 1 broken chocolate bar
- 1 pellet stevia/sugarfree

Directions
1. Blend ice, almond milk, protein powder and stevia/sugarfree.
2. Once done, add drinking chocolate and give it a whirl.
3. Fold in the whipped cream and gently stir in the broken chocolate and drink.
4. Sprinkle some nutmeg and cinnamon powder on top. Enjoy!

Coconut Almond Protein Joy Shake

Ingredients
- 1 cup fresh coconut cream (Malai)
- 1 ripe banana,
- 1 tbsp cocoa powder
- 2 tbsps shredded coconut
- 1 scoop whey protein supplement
- 200 ml soy milk
- 1 cup ice cubes
  Optional for garnish: Toasted dry coconut flakes, almonds

Directions
1. Blend all ingredients except the ones for garnishing.
2. Once blended, add almonds first and then dry coconut flakes as garnish and enjoy!

Chia Almond Spinach Shake

Ingredients
- 1 1/2 ripe bananas
- 1 1/2 cups Almond Milk
- 1 cup baby spinach leaves
- 2 tablespoons almond butter
- 2 tablespoons chia seeds
- 1 scoop vanilla flavor whey protein
- 1 cup ice
- 1 tablespoon grated chocolate bar

Directions
1. Blend everything except ice and chia seeds.
2. Once done, drop the ice cubes and chia seeds and give it a whirl.
3. Fold in the grated chocolate bar and serve.

Double Pina Colada Champion Smoothie

Ingredients
- 1 ½ cups crushed pineapple
- 1 medium ripe banana
- 1 cup thick Greek Yogurt (Dahi)
- 1 cup unsweetened almond milk
- 1 scoop protein powder (optional)
- 1 tablespoon almond butter
- Ice cubes

Directions
1. Blend pineapple till smooth.
2. Add everything and blend till smooth. Serve.

Coffee Peanut Protein Dream Smoothie

Ingredients
- 1 sachet instant coffee powder
- 1 ripe banana
- 1 tablespoon peanut butter
- 1 scoop whey protein powder
- 100 ml almond milk
- 2 tablespoon almond flakes
- 50 ml whipped cream
- 1 tablespoon grated chocolate bar
- 1 cup ice cubes

Directions
1. Blend everything except almond flakes, cream and chocolate till smooth.
2. Now fold in the whipped cream and gently slip in the grated chocolate bar. Serve.

Healthy Weight Gain Smoothie

Ingredients
- 2 Cups of coconut milk from a can
- 2 Bananas or Seasonal Mangoes
- 4 Tablespoons Peanut butter (or other nut butter)
- 1/4 cup pumpkin seeds
- 1/4 cup raisins
- 4 cups of spinach (optional)
- 1 avocado
- 1 teaspoon vanilla extract (optional)

Directions
1. Put all the ingredients together in a mixer and blend until they become a smooth paste.
2. Add ice to it as per your requirement to cool it down else you can make it and keep in fridge for later consumption.

Apple Dates Protein Shake

Ingredients
- 2 large red Kashmir Apples, cored
- 1 ripe banana
- 1 cup ice
- 1 cup unsweetened almond milk
- 1/2 cup Greek yogurt (Dahi)
- 1 teaspoon ground cinnamon
- 1 pinch of ground nutmeg
- 1 pinch of ground ginger
- 1 tiny pinch of ground cloves
- 1 scoop whey protein powder
- 2-3 Dates
- 1 tablespoon honey

Directions
1. Blend apples, banana, protein powder and Greek yoghurt till smooth.
2. Add almond milk, nutmeg, ginger, cinnamon, cloves, dates and honey and blend till smooth.
3. Add ice cubes and blend once again.

Banana Peanut Protein Shake

Ingredients
- 1 big ripe banana
- 1 scoop non-sweetened whey protein powder
- 100 ml full cream milk
- 4 tablespoons roasted peanut powder
- 2 tablespoons roasted peanuts, coarsely ground
- 1 pellet stevia/sugar-free
- 1 cup ice

Directions
1. Blend banana, whey protein powder and roasted peanut powder.
2. Next add milk, stevia pellet, ice cubes and blend again.
3. Now mix the coarsely ground peanuts and give it a whirl. The drink is ready.

Albana Blueberry Slurpee Smoothie

Ingredients

- 1 large banana
- Curd (dahi) 200 ml
- Almond butter 3 tablespoons
- Blueberries 100 grams
- Whey protein powder 1 scoops
- Almond milk 100 ml
- Dates, seeded and soaked in warm water for 10 minutes
- **Ice**

Directions

1. Blend all ingredients without ice first till smooth.
2. Once done, add ice and blend till the needed texture appears.

Strawberry Avocado Smoothie

Ingredients
- ¼ Cup milk
- ¾ Cup plain or vanilla yogurt
- 1 Whole banana
- 1 ½ Cup frozen strawberries
- ¼ avocado
- ¼ tsp Vanilla extract

Directions
1. Put milk and yogurt in the blender and to blend them together perfectly. IF the consistency is too thin, add more milk.
2. **Add peeled banana and avocado to it and blend further.**
3. Once it reaches a smooth consistency, add frozen strawberries along with vanilla extract and blend again.

Minty Chocolaty Creamy Shake

Ingredients
- Full-fat milk 400 ml
- I cup vanilla ice cream
- 1 bunch mint leaves
- Protein powder 2 full scoops
- 1 small banana
- Honey 1 tablespoon
- Milk cream 50 ml
- Ice cubes

Directions
1. Crush mint leaves coarsely. Add tablespoon of water and blend till you get a fine paste.
2. Squeeze all liquid out and discard the leaves. Add this liquid to all except ice cubes and give it a whirl.
3. Once done, add ice cubes and blend for another minute.

Sweet Cinnamon Smoothie

Ingredients
- 2 medium banana, sliced
- 1 tsp. nutmeg
- 1 tsp. cinnamon
- 1 tsp. vanilla extract
- 1 tsp. maple syrup
- Almond milk to fill line (unsweetened)
- Nuts as garnish (optional)
- Shredded Coconut as garnish (optional)

Directions
1. Put sliced banana and almond milk in mixer to blend together, add in rest of the ingredients except garnish and blend until all become smooth together.
2. **Add ice as per your requirement, blend again.**
3. Pour in glass and garnish with nuts and shredded coconut for added flavor.

Strawberry, Banana And Blueberry Smoothie

Ingredients
- 1/8 Cup milk
- 1/2 Cup plain yogurt
- 1 Whole banana
- 1/2 Cup frozen strawberries
- 1/2 Cup frozen blueberries
- Cinnamon, to taste

Directions
1. Pour milk in the blender, followed by yogurt and peeled banana.
2. **Blend until the banana is completely blended.**
3. Add frozen strawberry and blue berries along with a pinch of cinnamon to blend further.
4. You can either make a smooth paste or keep it coarse for some crunch in your smoothie.

Chocolate Coffee Blend

Ingredients
- Chocolate powder 1 tablespoon
- Instant Coffee powder 1 tablespoon
- Full-fat milk 400 ml
- Milk cream 100 ml
- Honey 2 tablespoons
- Chocolate ice cream 1 big cup
- Protein supplement 2 scoops
- Ice cubes

Directions
1. Blend coffee & chocolate powder, honey and cream.
2. Add ice cream and ice and blend well.

Part 2

Banana Smoothie

Ingredients:
- 2 Bananas
- ½ Cup of Vanilla Yogurt
- ½ Cup of Milk
- 2 tsp. of Honey
- Dash of Cinnamon
- 1 Cup of Ice

Directions:
1. Blend the ice.
2. Blend all of the ingredients into the ice.

Nutritional Information:
- Calories: 223
- Total Fat: 1g
- Saturated Fat: 0g
- Carbohydrates: 24g
- Protein: 6g

Banana And Strawberry Smoothie

Ingredients:
- 1 Banana
- 1 Cup of Strawberries
- ½ Cup of Vanilla Yogurt
- ½ Cup of Milk
- 2 tsp. of honey
- Dash of Cinnamon
- 1 Cup of Ice

Directions
1. Blend the ice in a blender or food processor.
2. Blend in the rest of the ingredients.

Nutritional Information:
- Calories: 235
- Total Fat: 2g
- Saturated Fat: 0g
- Carbohydrates: 21g
- Protein: 6.5g

Strawberry Shortcake Smoothie

Ingredients:
- 2 Cups of Strawberries
- 1 Cup of Pound Cake – Crumbled
- 1 ½ Cups of Milk
- 1 ½ Cup of Ice
- 1 tsp. of Sweetener
- Topping – Whipped Cream
- Topping – Chopped Strawberries

Directions:
1. Blend the ice.
2. Add in the milk, sweetener, cake, and 2 cups of strawberries.
3. Top it with chopped strawberries and whipped cream.

Nutritional Information:
- Calories: 274
- Total Fat: 4g
- Saturated Fat: 0g
- Carbohydrates: 21g
- Protein: 7g

Triple Blended Berry Smoothie

Ingredients:
- 1/3 Cup of Blackberries
- 1/3 Cup of Strawberries
- 1/3 Cup of Raspberries
- 1 Cup of Ice
- 1 Cup of Milk
- 1 tsp. of Sweetener

Directions:
1. Blend the ice.
2. Blend in the rest of the ingredients.

Nutritional Information:
- Calories: 215
- Total Fat: 1g
- Saturated Fat: 0g
- Carbohydrates: 20g
- Protein: 5g

Orange Raspberry Smoothie

Ingredients:
- 1 Cup of Orange Juice
- 1 Cup of Raspberries
- ½ Cup of Plain Yogurt
- 1 Cup of Ice
- 1 tsp. of Sweetener

Directions:
1. Blend the ice.
2. Blend the rest of the ingredients together.

Nutritional Information:
- Calories: 212
- Total Fat: 1g
- Saturated Fat: 0g
- Carbohydrates: 19g
- Protein: 4g

Mango Peach Banana Smoothie

Ingredients:
- 1 Cup of Peaches – Fresh or Frozen
- 1 Cup of Mango – Fresh or Frozen
- 1 Cup of Plain Yogurt
- 1 Cup of Ice
- ½ Banana
- 1 tsp. of Sweetener

Directions:
1. Blend in the ice.
2. Add in the rest of the ingredients and blend them together.

Nutritional Information:
- Calories: 210
- Total Fat: 1g
- Saturated Fat: 0g
- Carbohydrates: 18g
- Protein: 4g

Almond Honeydew Smoothie

Ingredients:
- 2 Cups of Honeydew Melon – Chopped
- 1 Cup of Almond Milk
- 1 Cup of Ice
- 2 tsp. of Honey

Directions:
1. Blend in the ice and the milk.
2. Blend in the rest of the ingredients.

Nutritional Information:
- Calories: 178
- Total Fat: 1g
- Saturated Fat: 0g
- Carbohydrates: 17g
- Protein: 4g

Cantaloupe Smoothie

Ingredients:
- 2 Cups of Cantaloupe – Chopped
- Juice from ½ Lime
- 3 Tbsp. of Sweetener
- ½ Cup of Water
- 1 Cup of Ice

Directions:
1. Blend the ice.
2. Blend in the rest of the ingredients.

Nutritional Information:
- Calories: 157
- Total Fat: 1g
- Saturated Fat: 0g
- Carbohydrates: 18g
- Protein: 5g

Apple And Carrots Smoothie

Ingredients:
- 1 Cup of Carrot Juice
- 1 Cup of Apple Juice
- 1 ½ Cups of Ice

Directions:
- Blend all of the ingredients together.

Nutritional Information:
- Calories: 124
- Total Fat: 1g
- Saturated Fat: 0g
- Carbohydrates: 16g
- Protein: 3g

Spa Cucumber Smoothie

Ingredients:
- 2 Medium Cucumbers
- Juice from 1 Lime
- ½ Cup of Water
- 1 Cup of Ice
- 3-4 Tbsp. of Honey

Directions:
1. Blend the ice and the water.
2. Blend in the rest of the ingredients.

Nutritional Information:
- Calories: 123
- Total Fat: 0g
- Saturated Fat: 0g
- Carbohydrates: 16g
- Protein: 3g

Cherry Vanilla Smoothie

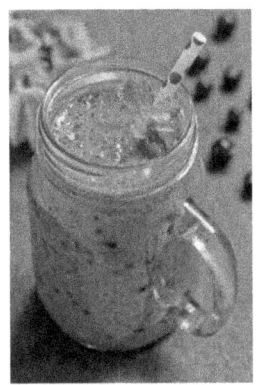

Ingredients:
- 1 ½ Cups of Cherries – Frozen
- 1 ¼ Cups of Milk
- 3 Tbsp. of Sweetener
- ½ tsp. of Vanilla
- ¼ tsp. of Almond Extract
- Dash of Salt
- 1 Cup of Ice

Directions:
1. Blend the ice, salt, and milk.
2. Blend in the rest of the ingredients.

Nutritional Information:
- Calories: 174
- Total Fat: 1g
- Saturated Fat: 0g
- Carbohydrates: 17g
- Protein: 4g

Grapefruit Smoothie

Ingredients:
- 2 Grapefruits
- 3-4 Tbsp. of Sweetener
- 1 Cup of Ice
- Dash of Cinnamon

Directions:
1. Blend the ice.
2. Add in the sweetener.
3. Add in the grapefruits.
4. Dash the top with cinnamon.

Nutritional Information:
- Calories: 113
- Total Fat: 0g
- Saturated Fat: 0g
- Carbohydrates: 4g
- Protein: 21g

Ginger Banana Smoothie

Ingredients:
- 1 Banana
- ¾ Cup of Vanilla Yogurt
- 1 Tbsp. of Honey
- ½ tsp. of Ginger – Grated

Directions:
1. Blend all of the ingredients together.

Nutritional Information:
- Calories: 157
- Total Fat: 1g
- Saturated Fat: 0g
- Carbohydrates: 34g
- Protein: 5g

Mango Shake

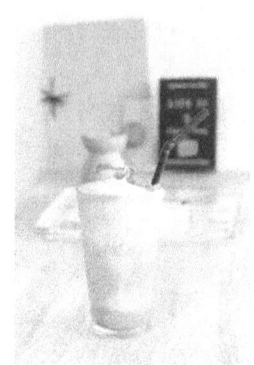

Ingredients:
- 1 Cup of Plain Yogurt
- 1 Cup of Ice
- 1 Large Mango – Peeled, Pitted, Chopped
- 1 Tbsp. of Sweetener
- Mint Leaf

Directions:
1. Put all of the ingredients, except for the mint, into your blender.
2. Blend it until it is blend.
3. Garnish is with the mint.

Nutritional Information:
- Calories: 178
- Total Fat: 2g
- Saturated Fat: 0g
- Carbohydrates: 21g

- Protein: 4g

Blue Raspberry Shake

Ingredients:
- 1 Cup of Blueberries – Frozen
- 1 Cup of Raspberries – Frozen
- 4-5 Tbsp. of Plain Yogurt
- ¾ Cup of Water
- ¼ Cup of Water
- 3 Tbsp. of Sweetener

Directions:
1. Put in the berries and the yogurt, then blend.
2. Blend in the rest of the ingredients.

Nutritional Information:
- Calories: 189
- Total Fat: 2g
- Saturated Fat: 0g
- Carbohydrates: 24g
- Protein: 7g

Mixed Berry Shake

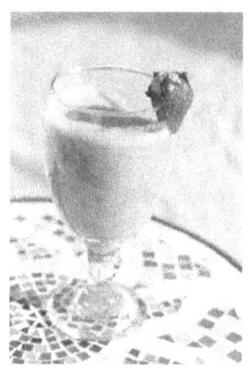

Ingredients:
- 2 Cups of Strawberries – Washed, Hulled
- ½ Cup of Cranberry Juice Cocktail
- 2 Tbsp. of Sweetener
- 1 Pint of Strawberry Yogurt – Frozen

Directions:
1. Combine all of the ingredients.
2. Garnish it with mint leaves.

Nutritional Information:
- Calories: 230
- Total Fat: 3g
- Saturated Fat: 1g
- Carbohydrates: 25g
- Protein: 7g

Buttermilk Strawberry Shake

Ingredients:
- 1 ½ Cups of Strawberries – Frozen
- 2 ½ Cups of Buttermilk – Low Fat
- ½ tsp. of Vanilla Extract
- 2 Tbsp. of Sweetener

Directions:
1. Place all of the ingredients in the blender.
2. Process them all until it is smooth.

Nutritional Information:
- Calories: 254
- Total Fat: 2g
- Saturated Fat: 0g
- Carbohydrates: 27g
- Protein: 9g

Mixed Berry Shake

Ingredients:
- 1 Quart Vanilla Ice Cream – Sugar Free
- 6 Ounces of Berries – Unsweetened, Frozen
- 2 Cups of Milk – Almond

Directions:
1. Combine in half of the sugar free ice cream, milk, and the berries.
2. Blend them until they are smooth.

Nutritional Information:
- Calories: 298
- Total Fat: 3g
- Saturated Fat: 0g
- Carbohydrates: 34g
- Protein: 8g

Cranberry Green Tea Shake

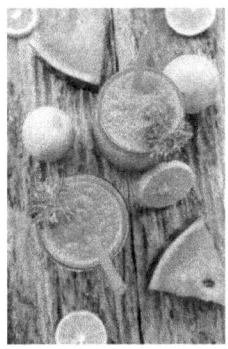

Ingredients:
- ½ Cup of Cranberries – Frozen
- ¼ Cup of Blueberries – Frozen
- ½ Cup of Blackberries – Frozen
- 5 Strawberries – Frozen
- 1 Banana
- ½ Cup of Green Tea – Cooled (Room Temperature)
- ¼ Cup of Soy Milk
- 2 Tbsp. of Honey

Directions:
1. Blend all of the ingredients together.
2. Drink immediately after.

Nutritional Information:
- Calories: 157
- Total Fat: 1g
- Saturated Fat: 0g
- Carbohydrates: 34g

- Protein: 5g

The Energy Shake

Ingredients:
- ½ Cup of Orange Juice
- 4-5 Strawberries – Hulled, Sliced
- ½ Banana
- ¼ Cup of Silken Tofu
- 1 Tbsp. of Honey
- 6 Cubes of Ice

Directions:
1. Blend the ice and the tofu.
2. Blend in the rest of the ingredients.

Nutritional Information:
- Calories: 156
- Total Fat: 0g
- Saturated Fat: 0g
- Carbohydrates: 21g
- Protein: 4g

Yogurt And Fruit Shake

Ingredients:
- 1 Cup of Cherries – Frozen
- 1 Cup of Yogurt – Plain
- 1 Cup of Pomegranate Cherry Juice
- 1 Can of Pineapple – Crushed, Keep the Juice
- 1 Banana – Peeled, Sliced

Directions:
1. Blend the ingredients together. Except for the banana slices.
2. Add the bananas to the top.

Nutritional Information:
- Calories: 215
- Total Fat: 2g
- Saturated Fat: 0g
- Carbohydrates: 21g
- Protein: 7g

Mango Blackberry Shake

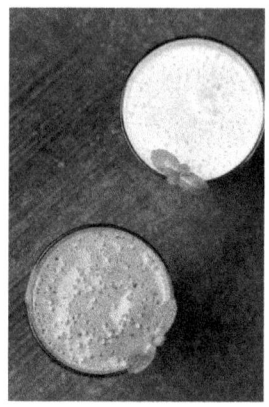

Ingredients:
- 1 ½ Cups of Blackberries – Frozen
- 1 Cup of Mango Slices
- 1 Cup of Tofu – Low Fat
- 1 Cup of Orange Juice
- 3 Tbsp. of Honey

Directions:
1. Blend all of the ingredients together.

Nutritional Information:
- Calories: 211
- Total Fat: 2g
- Saturated Fat: 0g
- Carbohydrates: 21g
- Protein: 4g

Strawberry Milk Shake

Ingredients:
- 8 Ounces of Strawberries – Stemmed, Sliced
- ½ tsp. of Vanilla Extract
- 1 Pint of Sugar Free Vanilla Ice Cream
- ¼ Cup of Milk

Directions:
1. Add in all of the ingredients.

Nutritional Information:
- Calories: 213
- Total Fat: 2g
- Saturated Fat: 0g
- Carbohydrates: 22g
- Protein: 6g

Fruit Yogurt Shake

Ingredients:
- 2 Cups of Sugar Free Vanilla Ice Cream
- 8 Ounces of Yogurt – Low Fat, Plain
- ½ Cup of Pineapple Orange Juice Concentrate – Thawed
- 2 Cups of Strawberries – Frozen
- 1 Banana – Chopped

Directions:
1. Blend in all of the ingredients.
2. Drink right after blending.

Nutritional Information:
- Calories: 215
- Total Fat: 1g
- Saturated Fat: 0g
- Carbohydrates: 24g
- Protein: 6g

Choco Cherry Smoothie

Total Time: 5 minutes
Serves: 2
Ingredients:
- 4 tbsp cocoa powder, unsweetened
- 2 cups cherries
- 2 cups almond milk, unsweetened
- 2 tbsp chia seeds
- 1/2 cup rolled oats
- 2 dates

Directions:
1. Add all ingredients into the blender and blend until smooth and creamy.

Nutritional Value (Amount per Serving):
- Calories 748
- Fat 60.7 g
- Carbohydrates 56.4 g
- Sugar 27.6 g
- Protein 11.8 g

Melon Mint Smoothie

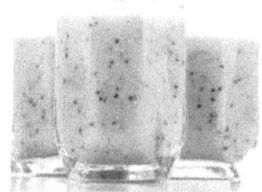

Total Time: 5 minutes
Serves: 2
Ingredients:
- 3 cups ripe honeydew melon
- 2 cup ice
- 20 mint leaves
- 5 tbsp lemon juice
- 1 1/3 cup plain vegan yogurt

Directions:
1. Add all ingredients into the blender and blend until smooth and creamy.
2. Serve and enjoy.

Nutritional Value (Amount per Serving):
- Calories 249
- Fat 2.7 g
- Carbohydrates 44.1 g
- Sugar 41.6 g
- Protein 11.0 g

Zinger Ginger Honeydew Smoothie

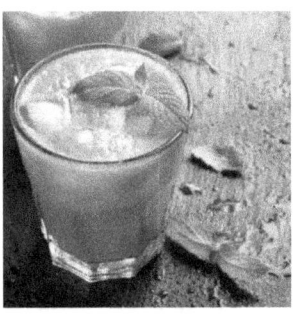

Total Time: 5 minutes
Serves: 2
Ingredients:
- 1 cup honeydew melon
- 1 inch ginger
- 1 ripe banana
- 1 cup watermelon
- 1 cup cantaloupe
- 1 cup almond milk

Directions:
1. Add all ingredients into the blender and blend until smooth.

Nutritional Value (Amount per Serving):
- Calories 408
- Fat 29.2 g
- Carbohydrates 39.9 g
- Sugar 28.9 g

- Protein 5.0 g

Guava Smoothie

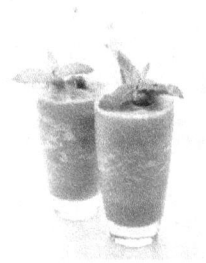

Total Time: 5 minutes
Serves: 2
Ingredients:
- 1 guava, sliced
- 4 tbsp coconut milk
- 1 cup fresh raspberries
- 1 cup pomegranate seeds
- 1/4 cup ice cubes

Directions:
1. Add all ingredients into the blender and blend until smooth.
2. Serve immediately and enjoy.

Nutritional Value (Amount per Serving):
- Calories 132

- Fat 8.0 g
- Carbohydrates 15.4 g
- Sugar 7.7 g
- Protein 2.6 g

Cranberry Banana Smoothie

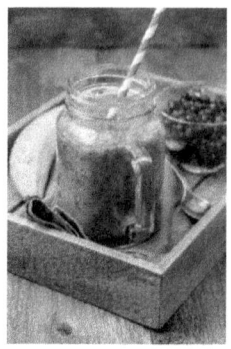

Total Time: 5 minutes
Serves: 2
Ingredients:
- 1 cup cranberries
- 1 banana
- 1 orange
- 1 cup almond milk, unsweetened
- 6 ice cubes

Directions:
1. Add all ingredients into the blender and blend until smooth and creamy.

Nutritional Value (Amount per Serving):
- Calories 402
- Fat 28.9 g
- Carbohydrates 35.9 g
- Sugar 21.8 g
- Protein 4.2 g

Apricot Berries Smoothie

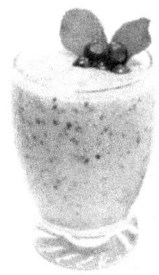

Total Time: 5 minutes
Serves: 2
Ingredients:
- 2 apricots, pitted
- 1 cup almond milk
- 1 cup mix berries
- 1 cup ice cubes

Directions:
1. Add all ingredients into the blender and blend until smooth and creamy.
2. Serve immediately and enjoy.

Nutritional Value (Amount per Serving):
- Calories 365
- Fat 29.1 g
- Carbohydrates 27.6 g
- Sugar 20.8 g
- Protein 3.7 g

Pear Blueberry Smoothie

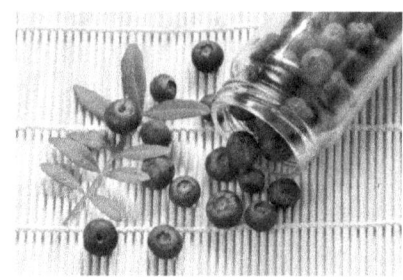

Total Time: 5 minutes
Serves: 4
Ingredients:
- 2 cups blueberries
- 1/2 cup water
- 1 pear, seeded and diced
- 1 1/2 cup plain vegan yogurt

Directions:
1. Add all ingredients into the blender and blend until smooth.

Nutritional Value (Amount per Serving):
- Calories 143
- Fat 1.4 g
- Carbohydrates 26.6 g
- Sugar 21.4 g
- Protein 5.9 g

Celery Cucumber Smoothie

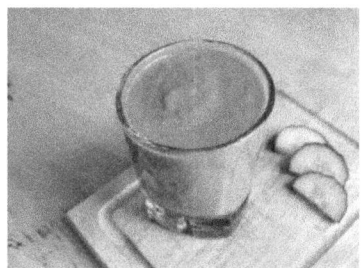

Total Time: 5 minutes
Serves: 2
Ingredients:
- 3 celery ribs
- 1 inch ginger
- 1 lemon juice
- 2 medium cucumbers

Directions:
1. Add all ingredients into the blender and blend until smooth.
2. Serve chilled and enjoy.

Nutritional Value (Amount per Serving):
- Calories 90
- Fat 0.7 g
- Carbohydrates 21.9 g
- Sugar 10.1 g
- Protein 3.9 g

Carrot Celery Ginger Smoothie

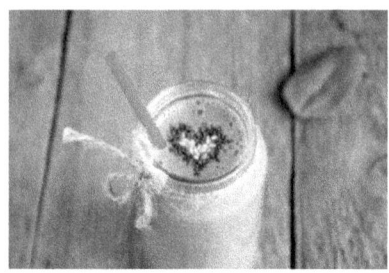

Total Time: 5 minutes
Serves: 2
Ingredients:
- 2 medium carrots
- 4 celery sticks
- 1 inch ginger piece
- 1 lemon juice
- 3 green apples

Directions:
1. Add all ingredients into the blender and blend until smooth.
2. Serve immediately and enjoy.

Nutritional Value (Amount per Serving):
- Calories 199
- Fat 0.6 g
- Carbohydrates 52.2 g
- Sugar 37.8 g

- Protein 1.4 g

Turmeric Pineapple Smoothie

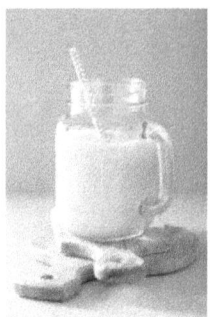

Total Time: 5 minutes
Serves: 2
Ingredients:
- 1 inch fresh turmeric piece, peeled
- 1 cup pineapple, cut into pieces
- 1 tsp vanilla extract
- 1 cup almond milk
- 1 banana
- 1 inch fresh ginger piece, peeled

Directions:
1. Add banana, ginger, pineapple and turmeric in blender and blend until smooth.
2. Now add vanilla extract and almond milk and blend again until smooth and creamy.
3. Serve immediately and enjoy.

Nutritional Value (Amount per Serving):
- Calories 376
- Fat 28.9 g

- Carbohydrates 31.2 g
- Sugar 19.6 g
- Protein 3.8 g

Cucumber Pineapple Grapefruit Smoothie

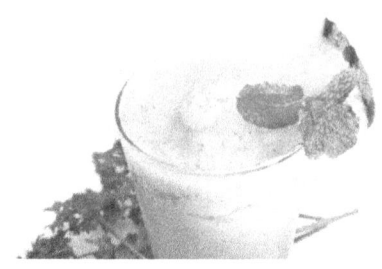

Total Time: 5 minutes
Serves: 2
Ingredients:
- 1 cucumber
- 1 cup pineapple chunks
- 1 grapefruit
- 1 inch ginger piece

Directions:
1. Add all ingredients into the blender and blend until smooth.

Nutritional Value (Amount per Serving):
- Calories 84
- Fat 0.3 g
- Carbohydrates 21.5 g
- Sugar 15.1 g
- Protein 1.8 g

Turmeric Pumpkin Smoothie

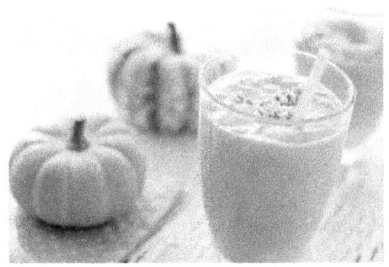

Total Time: 5 minutes
Serves: 2
Ingredients:
- 1 cup pumpkin
- 1 inch fresh turmeric piece
- 2 carrots, peeled
- 2 green apples
- 1/4 tsp cinnamon powder

Directions:
1. Add all ingredients into the blender and blend until smooth.

Nutritional Value (Amount per Serving):
- Calories 183
- Fat 0.7 g
- Carbohydrates 46.7 g
- Sugar 30.2 g
- Protein 2.5 g

Sweet Potato Ginger Smoothie

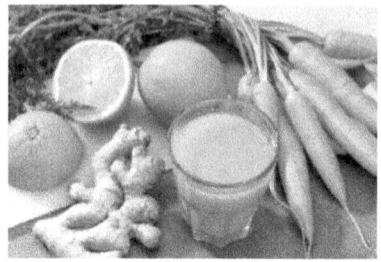

Total Time: 5 minutes
Serves: 2
Ingredients:
- 1 sweet potato
- 1 inch fresh ginger
- 2 carrots
- 1/2 cup pineapple chunks

Directions:
1. Add all ingredients into the blender and blend until smooth.

Nutritional Value (Amount per Serving):
- Calories 97
- Fat 0.3 g
- Carbohydrates 23.2 g
- Sugar 10.8 g
- Protein 1.9 g

Cucumber Ginger Smoothie

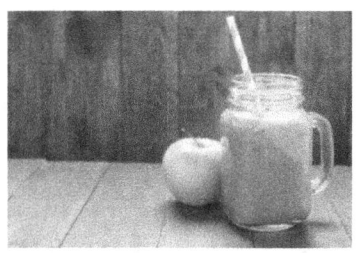

Total Time: 5 minutes
Serves: 2
Ingredients:
- 1/2 fennel
- 1 large cucumber
- 1 inch fresh ginger
- 1/4 lemon juice
- 2 green apples
- 4 celery ribs

Directions:
1. Add all ingredients into the blender and blend until smooth.

Nutritional Value (Amount per Serving):
- Calories 139
- Fat 0.6 g
- Carbohydrates 36.3 g
- Sugar 25.7 g
- Protein 1.6 g

Apple Peanut Butter Smoothie

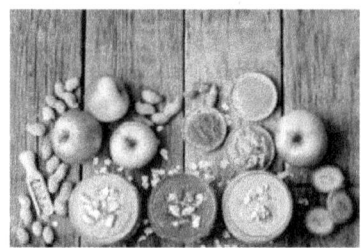

Total Time: 5 minutes
Serves: 4
Ingredients:
- 2 medium apples, diced
- 2 tbsp peanut butter
- 2 cups ice cubes
- 1 tsp cinnamon

Directions:
1. Add apple, peanut butter and ice cubes into the blender and blend until smooth and creamy.
2. Pour into the glasses and sprinkle with cinnamon on top.

Nutritional Value (Amount per Serving):
- Calories 106
- Fat 4.2 g
- Carbohydrates 17.4 g
- Sugar 12.4 g
- Protein 2.3 g

Chocolate Avocado Smoothie

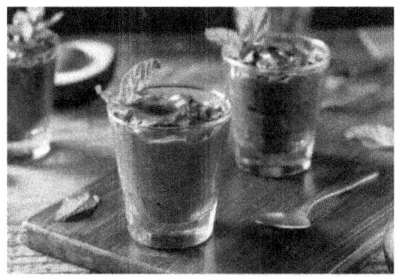

Total Time: 5 minutes
Serves: 2
Ingredients:
- 1/2 avocado, remove seed and scoop out
- 2 tbsp cocoa powder
- 1 1/2 cups almond milk, unsweetened
- 3 tbsp peanut butter
- 1 medium ripe banana

Directions:
1. Add all ingredients into the blender and blend until smooth and creamy.

Nutritional Value (Amount per Serving):
- Calories 738
- Fat 65.7 g
- Carbohydrates 39.8 g
- Sugar 20.1 g
- Protein 12.7 g

Hearty Spinach Lentil Soup

Serves: 4
Preparation Time: 35 minutes
Ingredients:
- 1 cup brown lentils, rinsed
- 5 cups spinach
- 4 cups vegetable stock
- 1/2 tsp thyme, dried
- 1/2 tsp turmeric
- 1 1/2 tsp ground cumin
- 2 tbsp garlic, minced
- 1/2 cup celery stalk, chopped
- 1 large carrot, peeled and diced
- 1 small onion, diced
- 2 tsp extra virgin olive oil
- 1/4 tsp pepper
- 1/2 tsp salt

Directions:
1. Add oil in instant pot then select sauté.
2. Once oil is hot then add onion, celery and carrots and sauté for 5 minutes.
3. Add thyme, turmeric, cumin, garlic, pepper and salt and stir for 1 minute.
4. Pour vegetable stock in pot. Stir well.
5. Add lentils and stir for minute.

6. Seal pot with lid and cook on high pressure for 12 minutes.
7. Release pressure using quick release method then open lid carefully.
8. Add spinach and stir well.
9. Serve warm and enjoy.

Nutritional Value (Amount per Serving):
- Calories 225
- Fat 3.3 g
- Carbohydrates 36.1 g
- Sugar 3.0 g
- Protein 14.3 g

Yummy Mac And Cheese

Serves: 4
Preparation Time: 20 minutes
Ingredients:
- 2 cups noodles, gluten free
- 4 tbsp vegan butter
- 2 cups cheddar cheese, shredded
- 1 cup heavy cream
- 1 cup vegetable broth
- Pepper
- Salt

Directions:
1. Add cream, noodles and vegetable broth in instant pot.
2. Seal pot with lid and cook for 7 minutes.
3. Release pressure using quick release method then open lid carefully.
4. Add butter, cheese and stir until melted.
5. Season with pepper and salt.
6. Serve and enjoy.

Nutritional Value (Amount per Serving):
- Calories 553 Fat 43.3 g Carbohydrates 21.9 g
- Sugar 0.8 g Protein 19.7 g

Creamy And Delicious Potato Mash

Serves: 6
Preparation Time: 15 minutes
Ingredients:
- 3 lbs potatoes, clean and diced
- 4 tbsp half and half
- 2 tbsp vegan butter
- 1 cup vegetable broth
- 1/4 tsp pepper
- 3/4 tsp salt

Directions:
1. Place steamer rack in the instant pot then pour vegetable broth.
2. Add potatoes and seal pot with lid.
3. Cook on manual high pressure for 8 minutes.
4. Release pressure using quick release method then open lid carefully.
5. Transfer potatoes in large mixing bowl and mash with masher.
6. Add half and half, butter, pepper and salt. Mix well until combine.
7. Serve hot and enjoy.

Nutritional Value (Amount per Serving):
- Calories 210 Fat 5.5 g
- Carbohydrates 36.3 g Sugar 2.8 g
- Protein 5.0 g

Kale Lentil Soup

Serves: 4
Preparation Time: 30 minutes
Ingredients:
- 2 kale stems, chopped
- 1 cup lentils
- 1 sweet potato, diced
- 1 bay leaf
- 4 cups vegetable stock
- 2 garlic cloves, minced
- 1 small onion, diced
- 2 carrots, diced
- 1 tsp salt

Directions:
1. Add in instant pot lentils, garlic, onion, carrots and sweet potato, bay leaf and vegetable stock.
2. Seal pot with lid and cook on manual high pressure for 20 minutes.
3. Release pressure using quick release method then open lid carefully.
4. Add chopped kale and salt in pot and stir for 2 to 3 minutes.
5. Serve and enjoy.

Nutritional Value (Amount per Serving):
- Calories 231
- Fat 0.8 g
- Carbohydrates 41.9 g

- Sugar 6.7 g
- Protein 14.4 g

Quick And Cheesy Pasta

Serves: 6
Preparation Time: 15 minutes
Ingredients:
- 1 lb pasta
- 1 cup half and half
- 15 oz broccoli, frozen
- 15 oz vegan cheddar cheese, shredded
- 4 cups water

Directions:
1. Add pasta, broccoli and water in instant pot and stir well.
2. Seal pot with lid and cook on high pressure for 4 minutes.
3. Release pressure using quick release method then open lid carefully.
4. Now select sauté function and add cheese and milk. Stir until cheese is melted.
5. Serve and enjoy.

Nutritional Value (Amount per Serving):
- Calories 580 Fat 30.1 g Carbohydrates 48.7 g
- Sugar 1.6 g Protein 29.4 g

Roasted Potatoes

Serves: 4
Preparation Time: 20 minutes
Ingredients:
- 1 1/2 lbs russet potatoes, cut into wedges
- 1 cup vegetable broth
- 1/4 tsp paprika
- 1 tsp garlic powder
- 1/2 tsp onion powder
- 4 tbsp olive oil
- 1/4 tsp pepper
- 1 tsp sea salt

Directions:
1. Add olive in instant pot and select sauté.
2. Once oil is hot then add potatoes and cook for 5 to 6 minutes.
3. Add remaining ingredients into the pot and mix well.
4. Seal pot with lid and cook for 6 minutes.
5. Release pressure using quick release method then open lid carefully.
6. Serve hot and enjoy.

Nutritional Value (Amount per Serving):
- Calories 251 Fat 14.5 g Carbohydrates 27.8 g
- Sugar 2.4 g Protein 4.2 g

Creamy Mushroom Risotto

Serves: 4
Preparation Time: 30 minutes
Ingredients:
- 2 cups Arborio rice
- 2 tsp extra virgin olive oil
- 1 tbsp vegan butter
- 1 cup vegan parmesan cheese, grated
- 4 cups vegetable stock
- 4 tbsp red wine
- 1 fresh thyme springs
- 3 cups mushrooms, sliced
- 1 medium onion, diced
- Pepper
- Salt

Directions:
1. Add olive oil in instant pot and select sauté.
2. Once oil is hot then adds onion and sauté until soften.
3. Add mushrooms and thyme and cook until soften.
4. Add rice and stir for minutes.
5. Pour vegetable stock and red wine in instant pot.
6. Season with pepper and salt.
7. Seal pot with lid and cook on manual high for 7 minutes.
8. Release pressure using quick release method then open lid carefully.

9. Add butter and cheese and stir until melted.
10. Serve hot and enjoy.

Nutritional Value (Amount per Serving):
- Calories 618
- Fat 18.3 g
- Carbohydrates 84.3 g
- Sugar 3.8 g
- Protein 27.4 g

Quick And Easy Green Beans

Serves: 2
Preparation Time: 10 minutes
Ingredients:
- 1 lb green beans
- 1 cup water
- Pepper
- Salt

Directions:
1. Pour water into the instant pot.
2. Add green beans in steamer basket and place basket in the pot.
3. Seal pot with lid and cook on manual high pressure for 1 minute.
4. Release pressure using quick release method then open lid carefully.
5. Season with pepper and salt.
6. Serve warm and enjoy.

Nutritional Value (Amount per Serving):
- Calories 70 Fat 0.3 g
- Carbohydrates 16.2 g Sugar 3.2 g
- Protein 4.1 g

Delicious Applesauce

Serves: 4
Preparation Time: 20 minutes
Ingredients:
- 3 lbs organic apples, peeled and diced
- 1/2 tsp ground nutmeg
- 1/4 cup water
- 1 cinnamon stick
- 1 tsp honey
- 1/8 tsp salt

Directions:
1. Add apples, nutmeg, water and cinnamon stick in instant pot.
2. Seal pot with lid and cook on high pressure for 5 minutes.
3. Release pressure using quick release method then open lid carefully.
4. Discard cinnamon stick and blend the sauce until you get desired consistency.
5. Add honey and salt to taste.

Nutritional Value (Amount per Serving):
- Calories 94
- Fat 0.4 g
- Carbohydrates 24.7 g
- Sugar 18.9 g
- Protein 0.5 g

Breakfast Rice Pudding
Serves: 6
Preparation Time: 30 minutes

Ingredients:
- 1 cup rice, rinse
- 1 tsp vanilla extract
- 1/8 tsp salt
- 4 tbsp maple syrup
- 3/4 cup coconut cream
- 1 1/4 cups water
- 2 cups almond milk

Directions:
1. Add rice, maple syrup, almond milk, water and salt in instant pot. Stir well.
2. Seal pot with lid and select porridge function. It takes 20 minutes.
3. Allow to release pressure naturally then open lid.
4. Add vanilla and coconut cream and stir until well combined.
5. Serve warm and enjoy.

Nutritional Value (Amount per Serving):
- Calories 402 Fat 26.5 g
- Carbohydrates 39.8 g
- Sugar 11.7 g
- Protein 4.7 g

Easy Steamed Brussels Sprouts

Serves: 4

Preparation Time: 10 minutes

Ingredients:
- 1 lb Brussels sprouts
- 4 tbsp pine nuts
- 1 cup water
- olive oil
- Pepper
- Salt

Directions:
1. Pour water into the instant pot.
2. Add Brussels sprouts in steamer basket and place basket in the pot.
3. Seal pot with lid and cook on manual high pressure for 3 minute.
4. Release pressure using quick release method then open lid carefully.
5. Season with pepper, salt and olive oil.
6. Sprinkle pine nuts and serve.

Nutritional Value (Amount per Serving):
- Calories 107 Fat 6.3 g Carbohydrates 11.4 g
- Sugar 2.8 g Protein 5.0 g

Garlic Chickpeas

Serves: 2
Preparation Time: 45 minutes
Ingredients:
- 1 cup dried chickpeas, rinse
- 2 bay leaves
- 3 garlic cloves
- 4 cups water

Directions:
1. Add chickpeas, bay leaves, garlic and water in instant pot.
2. Seal pot with lid and select bean function for 35 minutes.
3. Allow to release pressure naturally then open lid.
4. Serve warm and enjoy.

Nutritional Value (Amount per Serving):
- Calories 371
- Fat 6.1 g
- Carbohydrates 62.1 g
- Sugar 10.8 g
- Protein 19.6 g

Spinach Squash Risotto

Serves: 4
Preparation Time: 25 minutes
Ingredients:
- 1 1/2 cups Arborio rice
- 3 cups spinach
- 1/4 tsp oregano
- 1/2 tsp coriander
- 1 cup mushrooms
- 1/2 cup dry white wine
- 3 1/2 cups vegetable broth
- 1 1/2 cups butternut squash, peeled and diced
- 1 bell pepper, diced
- 2 garlic cloves, minced
- 1 small onion, chopped
- 1 tbsp olive oil
- 1/2 tsp pepper
- 1/2 tsp salt

Directions:
1. Add olive oil in instant pot and select sauté function.
2. Once oil is hot then add onion, squash, bell pepper and garlic and sauté for 5 minutes.
3. Add rice and stir until well combined.
4. Now add all remaining ingredients and mix well.
5. Seal pot with lid and cook on high for 5 minutes.
6. Release pressure using quick release method then open lid carefully.

7. Stir well and serve warm.

Nutritional Value (Amount per Serving):
- Calories 397
- Fat 5.4 g
- Carbohydrates 70.4 g
- Sugar 4.6 g
- Protein 11.3 g

Gluten Free Porridge

Serves: 2
Preparation Time: 25 minutes
Ingredients:
- 1/2 cup buckwheat groats, rinse
- 1/4 tsp vanilla extract
- 1/2 tsp cinnamon
- 2 tbsp raisins
- 1/2 banana, sliced
- 1 1/2 cups almond milk

Directions:
1. Add all ingredients into the instant pot and mix well to combine.
2. Seal pot with lid and cook on high pressure for 5 minutes.
3. Allow to release pressure naturally then open lid.
4. Stir well and serve warm.

Nutritional Value (Amount per Serving):
- Calories 571
- Fat 44.0 g
- Carbohydrates 45.6 g
- Sugar 15.8 g
- Protein 8.5 g

Apple Squash Soup

Serves: 6
Preparation Time: 25 minutes
Ingredients:
- 1 lb butternut squash, peeled and cubed
- 1 tbsp olive oil
- 4 cups vegetable broth
- 1 tsp ginger powder
- 1 medium apple, peeled and diced

Directions:
1. Add olive oil in instant pot and select sauté function.
2. Once oil is hot then add squash and cook for 5 minutes.
3. Now add all remaining ingredients and mix well.
4. Seal pot with lid and cook on high pressure for 10 minutes.
5. Release pressure using quick release method then open lid carefully.
6. Puree the soup using blender.
7. Serve warm and enjoy.

Nutritional Value (Amount per Serving):
- Calories 100 Fat 3.4 g
- Carbohydrates 14.8 Sugar 6.0 g
- Protein 4.1 g

Cilantro Lime Cauliflower Rice

Serves: 4
Preparation Time: 25 minutes
Ingredients:
- 1 lb cauliflower
- 1 fresh lime juice
- 4 tbsp fresh cilantro, chopped
- 1/4 tsp paprika
- 1/4 tsp turmeric
- 1/4 tsp cumin
- 1/2 tbsp parsley, dried
- 2 tbsp olive oil
- 1/4 tsp salt

Directions:
1. Wash cauliflower and cut into large florets.
2. Add all cauliflower florets into the steamer basket and place basket into the instant pot.
3. Pour 1 cup water into the instant pot.
4. Seal pot with lid and select manual for 1 minute.
5. Release pressure using quick release method then open lid carefully.
6. Transfer cauliflower into the plate.
7. Remove water from instant pot.
8. Add olive oil in pot and select sauté function.
9. Once oil is hot then add cooked cauliflower florets into the pot. Using masher break cauliflower.

10. Add paprika, turmeric, cumin, parsley and salt and stir for 2 minutes.
11. Transfer cauliflower rice in serving bowl and add lime juice.
12. Serve warm and enjoy.

Nutritional Value (Amount per Serving):
- Calories 90
- Fat 7.2 g
- Carbohydrates 6.3 g
- Sugar 2.7 g
- Protein 2.3 g

Refried Beans

Serves: 4
Preparation Time: 40 minutes
Ingredients:
- 1 cup dried pinto beans, rinsed
- 1/2 tsp cumin, ground
- 1 tsp oregano
- 2 cups water
- 2 cups vegetable broth
- 1/2 jalapeno, minced
- 2 garlic cloves, minced
- 1/2 onion, chopped
- 1/2 tbsp olive oil
- 1/4 tsp pepper

- 1/2 tsp salt

Directions:
1. Add olive oil in instant pot and select sauté function.
2. Once oil is hot then add onion, jalapeno and garlic and cook until soften.
3. Add all remaining ingredients and stir well.
4. Seal pot with lid and select manual for 30 minutes.
5. Allow to release pressure naturally then open lid.
6. Transfer bean mixture into the bowl and mash bean until smooth and creamy.
7. Season with pepper and salt.
8. Serve warm and enjoy.

Nutritional Value (Amount per Serving):
- Calories 212
- Fat 3.1 g
- Carbohydrates 32.9 g
- Sugar 2.0 g
- Protein 13.1 g

Creamy Potato Leek Soup

Serves: 4
Preparation Time: 25 minutes
Ingredients:
- 2 medium potatoes, peeled and diced
- 2 1/2 vegetable stock
- 1 bay leaf
- 1/2 tsp oregano, dried

- 1 leeks, sliced
- 1 tbsp olive oil
- 1/2 cup coconut milk
- 2 fresh thyme springs
- 3 garlic cloves, minced
- 1/2 tsp salt

Directions:
1. Add olive oil and leek in instant pot and select sauté for 1 minute.
2. Add salt and garlic and sauté for another 1 minute.
3. Add potatoes, vegetable stock, bay leaf, oregano and thyme. Stir.
4. Seal pot with lid and cook on high pressure for 8 minutes.
5. Release pressure using quick release method then open lid carefully.
6. Discard bay leaf and puree the soup using blender.
7. Add coconut milk and stir well.
8. Serve and enjoy.

Nutritional Value (Amount per Serving):
- Calories 190
- Fat 11.0 g
- Carbohydrates 22.1 g
- Sugar 3.2 g
- Protein 3.0 g

Plain Garlic Rice

Serves: 4
Preparation Time: 15 minutes
Ingredients:
- 1 cup rice, uncooked
- 1 1/2 cups water
- 1 tsp garlic, minced
- 1/8 tsp salt

Directions:
1. Rinsed rice and add in instant pot.
2. Add garlic, water and salt. Stir.
3. Seal pot with lid and select rice function.
4. Release pressure using quick release method then open lid carefully.
5. Fluff rice with fork and serve.

Nutritional Value (Amount per Serving):
- Calories 171
- Fat 0.4 g
- Carbohydrates 37.1 g
- Sugar 0.4 g
- Protein 3.1 g

Red Beans With Rice

Serves: 5
Preparation Time: 40 minutes
Ingredients:
- 1/2 lb dried red kidney beans
- 2 garlic cloves

- 1 celery stalks, diced
- 1 bell pepper, diced
- 1 onion, diced
- 1/4 tsp pepper
- 5 cups rice, cooked
- 3 1/2 cups water
- 1 bay leaf
- 1/4 tsp dried thyme
- 1/2 tsp salt

Directions:
1. Add all ingredients except rice in instant pot and mix well to combine.
2. Seal pot with lid and cook on high pressure for 25 minutes.
3. Allow to release pressure naturally then open lid.
4. Discard bay leaf from beans and stir well.
5. Serve with cooked rice and enjoy.

Nutritional Value (Amount per Serving):
- Calories 845
- Fat 1.9 g
- Carbohydrates 175.1 g
- Sugar 3.2 g
- Protein 24.0 g

Quick Sweet Potato Gratin

Serves: 4
Preparation Time: 20 minutes

Ingredients:
- 1 lb sweet potatoes, sliced
- 2 cups vegan cheddar cheese
- 1 cup vegan cream cheese
- 1 tbsp garlic powder
- 1/2 tbsp pepper
- 1 tsp chili powder
- 2 cups vegetable broth
- 3 garlic cloves, chopped
- 2 tbsp olive oil

Directions:
1. Add all ingredients into the instant pot except cheese.
2. Seal pot with lid and cook on high pressure for 4 minutes.
3. Allow to release pressure naturally then open lid.
4. Top with cheese and set pot with warm function for 5 minutes.
5. Serve and enjoy.

Nutritional Value (Amount per Serving):
- Calories 227
- Fat 8.0 g
- Carbohydrates 35.2 g
- Sugar 1.5 g
- Protein 4.8 g

Hot Ginger Carrot Soup

Serves: 4
Preparation Time: 6 hours 10 minutes
Ingredients:
- 5 medium carrots, shredded
- 1 tbsp garlic powder
- 1/2 tbsp pepper
- 3 cups vegetable broth
- 1 inch fresh ginger, peeled and chopped

Directions:
1. Add all ingredients into the instant pot.
2. Seal pot with lid and cook on low for 6 hours.
3. Using blender puree the soup until smooth and creamy.
4. Serve hot and enjoy.

Nutritional Value (Amount per Serving):
- Calories 69
- Fat 1.1 g
- Carbohydrates 10.2 g
- Sugar 4.8 g
- Protein 4.7 g

Sweet Brown Rice

Serves: 2
Preparation Time: 15 minutes
Ingredients:
- 1 cup brown rice
- 2 tbsp maple syrup

- 1 1/2 cups water

Directions:
1. Add all ingredients into the instant pot.
2. Seal pot with lid and cook on high for 8 minutes.
3. Allow to release pressure naturally then open lid.
4. Serve warm and enjoy.

Nutritional Value (Amount per Serving):
- Calories 396
- Fat 2.6 g
- Carbohydrates 85.8 g
- Sugar 11.9 g
- Protein 7.1 g

Cilantro Avocado Rice

Serves: 3
Preparation Time: 25 minutes
Ingredients:
- 1 cup rice
- 1/2 avocado, flesh
- 1 1/4 cups vegetable broth
- 1/4 cup green hot sauce
- 1/2 cup fresh cilantro, chopped
- Pepper
- Salt

Directions:
1. Add vegetable broth and rice in instant pot.

2. Seal pot with lid and cook on high pressure for 3 minutes.
3. Allow to release pressure naturally then open lid.
4. Add green sauce, avocado and cilantro in blender and blend until smooth.
5. Add avocado mixture into the rice and mix well.
6. Season with pepper and salt.
7. Serve and enjoy.

Nutritional Value (Amount per Serving):
- Calories 311 Fat 7.4 g Carbohydrates 52.8 g
- Sugar 0.7 g
- Protein 7.2 g

Mushroom Barley Risotto

Serves: 4
Preparation Time: 40 minutes
Ingredients:
- 1 cup barley
- 2 cups mushrooms, sliced and sautéed
- 1/4 cup white wine
- 3 cups vegetable stock
- 2 garlic cloves, minced
- 1 onion, chopped
- 1 cup dry wild mushrooms, soaked and sliced

- 4 tbsp cashew paste
- 1/4 cup parsley, chopped
- 1 tsp fresh rosemary
- 1 tbsp olive oil
- Pepper
- Salt

Directions:
1. Add olive oil in instant pot and select sauté.
2. Once oil is hot then add garlic, onion, pepper and salt, stir well and sauté for 3 minutes.
3. Add soaked mushrooms, rosemary and thyme. Stir.
4. Add white wine and cook until liquid absorb.
5. Add vegetable stock and barley in pot. Stir.
6. Seal pot with lid and cook on high pressure for 15 minutes.
7. Release pressure using quick release method then open lid carefully.
8. Add sautéed mushrooms, parsley and cashew paste, stir until combine.
9. Serve and enjoy.

Nutritional Value (Amount per Serving):
- Calories 232
- Fat 4.9 g
- Carbohydrates 39.8 g
- Sugar 2.7 g
- Protein 8.1 g

Delicious Sweet Potato Casserole

Serves: 4
Preparation Time: 30 minutes
Ingredients:
- 2 sweet potatoes, peeled and cut into 1/4 inch slices
- 1/3 cup pecans, chopped
- 2 tbsp heavy cream
- 3 tbsp coconut milk
- 1/8 tsp nutmeg
- 1/2 tsp cinnamon
- 1/2 tsp vanilla extract
- 2 tbsp vegan butter
- 1 tbsp flour
- 1/3 cup coconut sugar
- 1 tbsp vegan butter
- 1/2 cup raw cane sugar

Directions:
1. Pour 1 cup water into the instant pot and place sliced potatoes onto the basket.
2. Place steamer basket on the bottom of instant pot.
3. Seal pot with lid and cook on high pressure for 8 minutes.
4. Release pressure using quick release method then open lid carefully.
5. Transfer potatoes in large bowl.

6. Add 1/2 cup coconut sugar, 2 tbsp butter, nutmeg, vanilla and cinnamon. Mix well and beat with blender until smooth.
7. Add coconut milk and cream. Mix well to combine.
8. Pour mixture into casserole dish.
9. Combine together 1 tbsp butter, flour, 1/3 cup raw cane sugar and pecans. Sprinkle evenly over the top of casserole.
10. Place trivet in instant pot.
11. Pour 1 cup water in pot and place casserole dish on trivet.
12. Seal pot with lid and cook on high pressure for 13 minutes.
13. Release pressure using quick release method then open lid carefully.
14. Serve and enjoy.

Nutritional Value (Amount per Serving):
- Calories 334
- Fat 14.3 g
- Carbohydrates 50.9 g
- Sugar 17.7 g
- Protein 2.4 g

Millet Breakfast Porridge

Serves: 4
Preparation Time: 25 minutes
Ingredients:
- 2 cup millet flakes
- 1 tsp ground cinnamon
- 1 tbsp vegan butter
- 1 tsp vanilla extract
- 1 tbsp coconut oil
- 3 tbsp maple syrup
- 2 cups heavy cream
- 1 cup water

Directions:
1. Add all ingredients into the instant pot and mix well.
2. Seal pot with lid and cook on high pressure for 2 minutes.
3. Allow to release pressure naturally then open lid carefully.
4. Stir well and serve.

Nutritional Value (Amount per Serving):
- Calories 280 Fat 25.6 g
- Carbohydrates 12.3 g Sugar 9.1 g
- Protein 1.2 g

Potato Carrot Corn Chowder

Serves: 4
Preparation Time: 25 minutes
Ingredients:
- 1 large potato, diced
- 1 cup fresh corn
- 1 garlic clove, minced
- 1 celery stalk, chopped
- 1 carrot, peeled and chopped
- 1 onion, chopped
- 1 1/2 tbsp cornstarch
- 3 cups vegetable stock
- 1/2 tsp fresh thyme
- 1 tsp olive oil
- 1/4 tsp pepper
- 1/2 tsp salt

Directions:
1. Add olive oil in instant pot and select sauté function.
2. Once oil is hot then add garlic, celery, onion and carrots and sauté for 3 minutes.
3. Add stock, potatoes, corn and seasoning. Stir.
4. Seal pot with lid and cook on high pressure for 4 minutes.
5. Allow to release pressure naturally then open lid.
6. Combine together water and cornstarch. Whisk in potato mixture.
7. Set pot on sauté mode for 2 minutes.
8. Stir well and serve.

Nutritional Value (Amount per Serving):
- Calories 159

- Fat 1.8 g
- Carbohydrates 33.7 g
- Sugar 3.8 g
- Protein 4.0 g

Sweet And Spicy Spaghetti

Serves: 6
Preparation Time: 15 minutes
Ingredients:
- 1 lb spaghetti
- 2 tsp dried basil
- 2 garlic cloves, minced
- 1 onion, chopped
- 2 tbsp olive oil
- 2 1/2 cups water
- 15 oz tomato sauce
- 3 oz tomato paste
- 28 oz tomatoes, chopped
- 1/4 tsp red chili flakes
- 1 tsp brown sugar
- 2 tsp dried parsley
- 1 tsp dried oregano
- 1/4 tsp pepper
- 1/2 tsp salt

Directions:
1. Add olive oil in instant pot and select sauté function.
2. Once oil is hot then add onion and sauté for 2 minutes.

3. Add garlic and sauté for minute.
4. Now add all remaining ingredients and mix well until combine.
5. Seal pot with lid and cook on high pressure for 5 minutes.
6. Allow to release pressure naturally then open lid.
7. Stir and serve.

Nutritional Value (Amount per Serving):
- Calories 325
- Fat 6.8 g
- Carbohydrates 56.9 g
- Sugar 10.1 g
- Protein 11.6 g

Pea Corn Herbed Risotto

Serves: 4
Preparation Time: 15 minutes
Ingredients:
- 1 cup Arborio rice
- 1/2 cup sweet corn
- 1/2 cup peas
- 1 red pepper, diced
- 3 cups vegetable stock
- 1 tbsp extra virgin olive oil
- 2 garlic cloves, minced
- 1 onion, chopped
- 1 tsp mix herbs

- 1/4 pepper
- 1/2 tsp salt

Directions:
1. Add olive oil in instant pot and select sauté function.
2. Add onion and garlic and sauté for 4 minutes.
3. Add rice and mix well to combine.
4. Now add all remaining ingredients and stir well.
5. Seal pot with lid and cook on high pressure for 8 minutes.
6. Release pressure using quick release method then open lid carefully.
7. Stir and serve.

Nutritional Value (Amount per Serving):
- Calories 260
- Fat 4.1 g
- Carbohydrates 50.2 g
- Sugar 4.9 g
- Protein 5.7 g

Healthy Breakfast Quinoa

Serves: 6
Preparation Time: 15 minutes
Ingredients:
- 1 1/2 cups quinoa, uncooked and rinsed
- 2 tbsp maple syrup
- 2 1/4 cups water
- 1/2 tsp vanilla extract

- 1/4 tsp ground cinnamon
- Berries and slice almonds for topping

Directions:
1. Add water, quinoa, vanilla, maple syrup, cinnamon and salt in instant pot. Mix well.
2. Seal pot with lid and cook on high pressure for 1 minute.
3. Allow to release pressure naturally then open lid.
4. Stir and serve sliced almonds and berries.

Nutritional Value (Amount per Serving):
- Calories 176
- Fat 2.5 g
- Carbohydrates 32.0 g
- Sugar 4.1 g
- Protein 6.1 g

Quick Apple Crisp

Serves: 4
Preparation Time: 15 minutes
Ingredients:
- 4 apples, peeled and chopped
- 1/2 tsp salt
- 1/2 cup water
- 1/2 tsp nutmeg
- 3/4 cup rolled oats
- 1/4 cup coconut sugar
- 1/4 cup flour

- 4 tbsp vegan butter
- 1 tbsp maple syrup
- 2 tsp ground cinnamon

Directions:
1. Add apples in the instant pot.
2. Sprinkle with nutmeg and cinnamon. Add maple syrup and water. Mix well.
3. Melt butter in bowl and mix together melted butter, brown sugar, salt, oats and flour. Add spoonful on top of apples mixture.
4. Seal pot with lid and cook on manual high pressure for 8 minutes.
5. Allow to release pressure naturally then open lid.
6. Serve with ice-cream and enjoy.

Nutritional Value (Amount per Serving):
- Calories 334
- Fat 13.1 g
- Carbohydrates 54.9 g
- Sugar 31.1 g
- Protein 3.6 g

Garlic Tomato Beans

Serves: 4
Preparation Time: 25 minutes
Ingredients:
- 2 tbsp extra virgin olive oil
- 1 onion, chopped

- 1 lb pinto beans, soaked overnight
- 1/2 tsp dried sage
- 1/2 tsp dried oregano
- 1/2 tsp garlic powder
- 14 oz tomatoes, chopped
- 4 cups water
- Pepper
- Salt

Directions:
1. Add 1 tbsp olive oil in instant pot and select sauté function.
2. Once oil is hot then add onion and cook about 5 minutes.
3. Add soaked pinto beans, water and remaining olive oil in instant pot and seal pot with lid then select bean/ chili function.
4. Release the pressure using quick release method then open lid carefully.
5. Add tomatoes, sage, oregano, garlic powder, pepper and salt. Mix well to combine.
6. Select sauté mode on low set timer for 15 minutes.
7. Serve warm and enjoy.

Nutritional Value (Amount per Serving):
- Calories 485
- Fat 8.6 g
- Carbohydrates 78.0 g
- Sugar 6.4 g
- Protein 25.7 g

Creamy Squash And Apple Mash

Serves: 4
Preparation Time: 20 minutes
Ingredients:
- 1 lb butternut squash, cut into cubes
- 2 medium apples, cored and sliced
- 1/4 tsp ground cinnamon
- 1/8 tsp ginger
- 1 cup water
- 2 tbsp coconut oil
- 1 onion, sliced
- 1/4 tsp salt

Directions:
1. Pour 1 cup water into the instant pot and place steamer basket inside the pot.
2. Combine together apples, onion and butternut squash in steamer basket.
3. Sprinkle salt over the apple and butternut squash.
4. Seal pot with lid and select manual high pressure for 8 minutes.
5. Release pressure using quick release method then open lid carefully.
6. Transfer apple and squash mixture into the large bowl.
7. Using masher mash the apple and squash.
8. Add coconut oil, cinnamon and ginger in bowl and mix well to combine.

9. Serve and enjoy.

Nutritional Value (Amount per Serving):
- Calories 170
- Fat 7.2 g
- Carbohydrates 28.4 g
- Sugar 13.2 g
- Protein 1.8 g

Split Pea Curry

Serves: 4
Preparation Time: 20 minutes
Ingredients:
- 1 cup dried split peas
- 1 tomato, chopped
- 1/4 cup plain yogurt
- 1 tbsp olive oil
- 1 red chili pepper, diced
- 1 tsp vegan butter
- 1 onion, chopped
- 1 garlic clove, minced
- 1/2 tsp garam masala
- 1/4 tsp turmeric powder
- 1/2 tsp dry mustard
- 2 tsp ginger, grated
- 2 cups water

- 2 tbsp corianders, chopped
- 1/4 tsp asafetida

Directions:
1. Rinse split peas.
2. Add olive oil in instant pot and select sauté.
3. Once oil is hot then add asafetida and dry mustard. Stir for 50 seconds.
4. Add onions and garlic and sauté until onion soften.
5. Add all other ingredients except garam masala, corianders and salt in pot.
6. Seal pot with Lid and cook on manual high pressure for 10 minutes.
7. Release pressure using quick release method then Open lid carefully.
8. Add garam- masala and salt and stir well.
9. Garnish with chopped corianders and serve with rice.

Nutritional Value (Amount per Serving):
- Calories 237
- Fat 5.6 g
- Carbohydrates 35.1 g
- Sugar 6.0 g
- Protein 13.6 g

www.ingramcontent.com/pod-product-compliance
Lightning Source LLC
Chambersburg PA
CBHW071442070526
44578CB00001B/200